Mathematics for Veterinary Medical Technicians

Mathematics for Veterinary Medical Technicians

A Text/Workbook with Applications

Edward M. Stumpf
Frederick R. Fritz
William W. Bradford
Central Carolina Community College

Carolina Academic Press
Durham, NC

ISBN 0-89089-343-8 LCCN 2003107753

Carolina Academic Press
700 Kent Street
Durham, North Carolina 27701
Telephone (919) 489-7486
Fax (919) 493-5668
www.cap-press.com

Printed in the United States of America

Contents

Acknowledgments

We would like to thank all who contributed in the writing and production of this text. In particular, Doctor Paul Porterfield and Doctor Cindy Kuder, the Veterinary Technology Department of Central Carolina Community College and all the Veterinary Medical students who used early versions of the text and offered suggestions for improvement and corrections, and Donny Campbell for his help with drawings.

Introduction

This text provides a one-semester course in the basics of mathematics needed for Veterinary Technicians and Assistants. The course covers fractions, decimals and percentage without the use of calculators as is the case on most State Board Exams. The language is designed to be readable and in terms of everyday usage rather than formal and strict mathematical terms.

In addition to basic mathematical computations, several chapters are devoted to dosage and concentration problems in the English, Metric and Avoirdupois systems of measurement. An introduction to graphs and graphing techniques is included as well as basic statistics.

The workbook style of the text allows students freedom to move at a pace that ensures mastery of the material as well as flexibility for covering topics in any prescribed manner. You should read the material, study the examples, and work all the exercises in a particular exercise set before checking the answers which are provided in the Answer Keys.

In many programs, this may be the only math course students are required to take. If this is one of your early course offerings, you will find the material valuable and useful for other course requirements such as chemistry and clinical practices.

It is our hope that you will find the material useful and pertinent. If you have comments or suggestions please contact me at:

Ed Stumpf
c/o Marketing
Carolina Academic Press
700 Kent Street
Durham, NC 27701

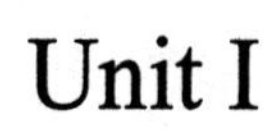

Unit I

Chapter 1

Roman Numerals

Objectives

Upon completion, the student must be able to do the following:

- **Write Roman Numerals for Arabic numerals from 1 to 30.**
- **Write Arabic numerals for Roman numerals from 1 to 30.**
- **Write selected Roman numerals for Arabic numerals greater than 30.**
- **Write selected Arabic numerals from Roman numerals greater than 30.**

Two systems of numbers are used by physicians in the clinic and for prescribing drugs – the Arabic and the Roman. The Arabic system utilizes the numerals 1, 2, 3, 4, 5, 6, 7, 8, 9, 0. It is the system commonly used in mathematics. All numerical values may be expressed by combinations of these ten symbols. The Arabic system is used to express weights and measures of the metric system and fractional units of the apothecaries' system.

The various Roman numerals used are:

Arabic	Roman
1	I or i
5	V or v
10	X or x
50	L or l
100	C or c
500	D or d
1000	M or m

In the Roman system, seven letters are used as symbols for numerals (indicated above). These letters are combined to express numerical values. When the apothecary system is used, whole units are expressed by Roman numerals. Lowercase or uppercase (capital) letters may be used to express Roman numerals, but it is customary to use small letters to indicate values of apothecary units. Cases are not mixed. Values over 30 are seldom used in medical practice; however, it is helpful to be familiar with Roman numerals above 30. The lower-case Roman numeral i (1) is always written with a dot over it to avoid confusion with the lower-case Roman letter l (50). In modern times, the use of lowercase Roman numerals has declined, particularly for values greater than fifty.

When reading or writing Roman numerals, pay attention to the position of the lesser values of numerals, such as I or V, in relation to the numerals of greater value, such as X or L.

Rules for Reading or Writing Roman Numerals

1) When a numeral is followed by the same numeral or by one of lesser value, the values of the numerals are added:

ii or II	xiii or XIII	xv or XV
means 1 + 1 or 2	means 10 + 1 + 1 + 1 or 13	means 10 + 5 or 15

2) When a numeral is written before one of greater value, the lesser value is subtracted from the greater one.

iv or IV	ix or IX
means 5 – 1 or 4	means 10 – 1 or 9

3) When a numeral is written between two or more numerals of greater value, its value is subtracted from the sum of the others in the numeral.

xix or XIX	xxxix or XXXIX
means 10 + 10 – 1 = 20 – 1 or 19	means 10 + 10 + 10 + 10 – 1 = 40 – 1 or 39

OR

The value of the preceding numerals of greater value are first determined. Then the value of the last two numerals are determined. The two groups are then added together to find the total value.

xix or XIX	xxxix or XXXIX	xxiv or XXIV
10 + 9 = 19	10 + 10 + 10 + 9 = 30 + 9 = 39	10 + 10 + 4 = 20 + 4 = 24

4) Numerals are used a maximum of three times in succession.

iii or III	xx or XX
means 1 + 1 + 1 is 3	means 10 + 10 = 20

5) I (or i) can precede only V(v) or X(x)
X (x) can precede only L or C
C can precede only D or M

6) Numerals of larger values use the same rules in the same order — the numbers are just more complex.

MCXXIV
M C XX IV
1000 + 100 + 20 + 4 =
1124

MCMXXIV
M CM XX IV
1000 + 900 + 20 + 4 =
1924

MCMXLIX
M CM XL IX
1000 + 900 + 40 + 9 =
1949

MMCMLXXXVIII
MM CM LXXX VIII
2000 + 900 + 80 + 8 =
2988

On the following page is a chart with some of the more common Roman numerals and their Arabic equivalents.

NUMERALS 1 - 30

Arabic	Roman	Arabic	Roman
1	I or i	10+5+1=16	XVI or xvi
1+1	II or ii	10+5+1+1=17	XVII or xvii
1+1+1	III or iii	10+5+1+1+1=18	XVIII or xviii
5–1=4	IV or iv	10+10-1=19	XIX or xix
5	V or v	10+10=20	XX or xx
5+1=6	VI or vi	10+10+1=21	XXI or xxi
5+1+1=7	VII or vii	10+10+1+1=22	XXII or xxii
5+1+1+1=8	VIII or viii	10+10+1+1+1=23	XXIII or xxiii
10 – 1=9	IX or ix	10+10+5-1=24	XXIV or xxiv
10	X or x	10+10+5=25	XXV or xxv
10+1=11	XI or xi	10+10+5+1=26	XXVI or xxvi
10+1+1=12	XII or xii	10+10+5+1+1=27	XXVII or xxvii
10+1+1+1=13	XIII or xiii	10+10+5+1+1+1=28	XXVIII or xxviii
10+5–1=14	XIV or xiv	10+10+10–1=29	XXIX or xxix
15	XV or xv	10+10+10=30	XXX or xxx

Practice Set I - 1 Convert to Roman or Arabic numerals as appropriate

1) __________ XX

2) 15 __________

3) 30 __________

4) __________ XXVI

5) 9 __________

6) __________ XXIII

7) 29 __________

8) __________ xix

9) 8 __________

10) 16 __________

11) __________ MCLXXIX

12) 1973 __________

13) __________ LXIV

14) __________ XCIX

15) 1975 __________

16) __________ CDXLVIII

17) 112 __________

18) 49 __________

19) __________ MMMCCCXXXIII

20) 2222 __________

Chapter 2

Introduction to Fractions

Objectives

Upon completion, the student must be able to do the following:

- **Name the parts of a fraction.**
- **Name all types of fractions.**
- **Reduce and express fractions in lowest terms.**
- **Change improper fractions to mixed numbers and vice versa.**

The actual measurement of many of the quantities with which we deal in the lab, in the home and in business force us to realize that the use of whole numbers alone is not sufficient to represent all this information. We simply are forced into using fractional measurements. Veterinary assistants especially should be able to solve problems involving fractions.

The parts of a fraction are called terms. In any common fraction there are two terms — Numerator and Denominator. The *Denominator* is the number written below the line of the fraction. It shows into how many equal parts the unit has been divided. In the following fractions, which number is the denominator:

a. $\frac{2}{3}$ b. $\frac{3}{7}$ c. $\frac{2}{5}$ d. $\frac{1}{16}$

If your answers are 3, 7, 5, 16, then you are correct. Fraction "a" indicates a whole unit has been divided into how many equal parts? _____. (If you selected 3, you are correct.)

The *Numerator* is the number written above the line of the fraction and shows how many equal parts there are of the unit. In the following fractions, which number is the Numerator?

a. $\frac{1}{16}$ b. $\frac{7}{12}$ c. $\frac{1}{2}$ d. $\frac{3}{8}$

Your answers should read: 1, 7, 1, 3

The following figures have been divided into equal parts. A certain number of these parts have been shaded. Write the fraction that indicates what part of each figure is shaded.

(a) 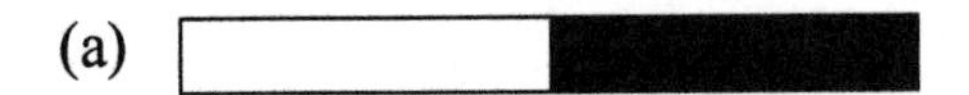

(b) 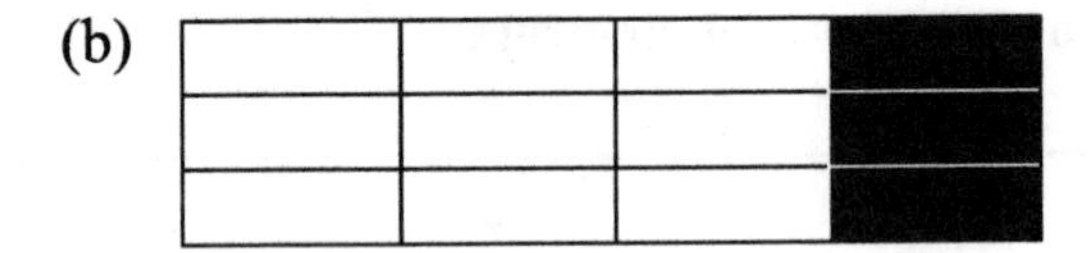

(c) 

(d) 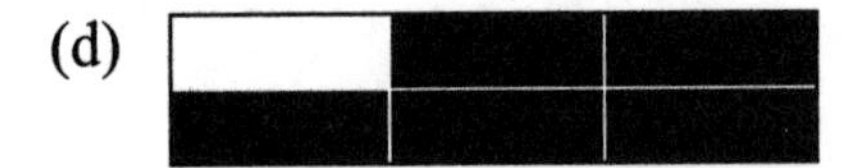

Your answer for "a" should be $^1/_2$. The denominator 2 indicates the units have been divided into two equal parts. The numerator 1 indicates that only one of the equal parts has been shaded. The correct answer for "b", "c", and "d" is $^3/_{12}$, $^3/_4$ and $^5/_6$.

In Exercise II-1 express your answer in fractions. Be sure to check your answers and correct any incorrect work.

Practice Set II - 1

1) List the shaded parts of each figure in terms of a fraction:

(a) 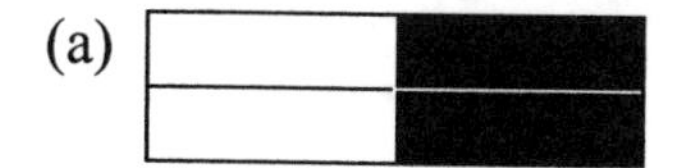 (b) 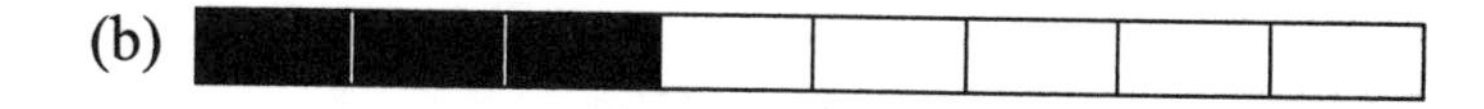

(c) 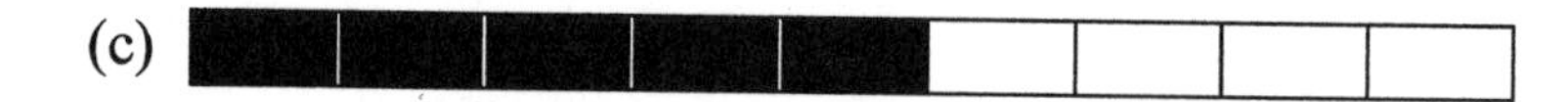 (d) 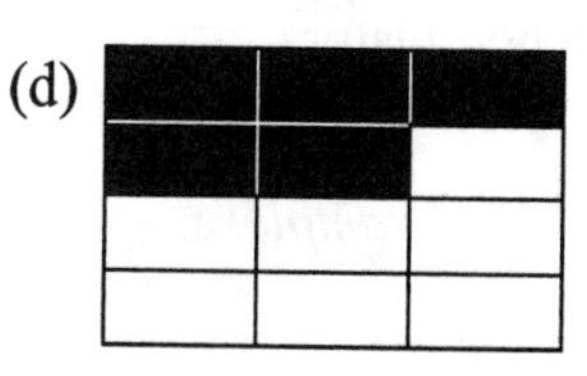

2) Express each of the following as a fraction of a foot (12" in a ft.):

a. 1 in. ______ b. 5 in. _____ c. 11 in. _____ d. 7 in. _____

3) There are 36 inches in a yard. Express each of these as fractions of a yard:

a. 1 in. _____ b. 35 in. _____ c. 13 in. _____ d. 19 in. _____

4) Express each of the following as fractions of an hour:

a. 7 min. _____ b. 13 min. _____ c. 30 min. _____ d. 45 min. _____

5) Express each of the problems shown as fractions of a dollar:

a. 12 cents ____ b. 37 cents _____ c. 50 cents _____ d. 99 cents _____

Common Fractions are fractions whose numerators and denominators are whole numbers.

Example: a. $\frac{1}{2}$ b. $\frac{16}{9}$ c. $\frac{2}{3}$ d. $\frac{5}{4}$

Proper Fractions are fractions which are less than one, that is whose numerators are less than the denominators.

Example: a. $\frac{1}{2}$ b. $\frac{1}{3}$ c. $\frac{16}{19}$ d. $\frac{8}{9}$

Improper Fractions have numerators which are equal to or larger than the denominators.

Example: a. $\frac{11}{6}$ b. $\frac{24}{23}$ c. $\frac{4}{3}$ d. $\frac{8}{5}$

Mixed Numbers are whole numbers and fractions.

Example: a. $1\frac{5}{6}$ b. $1\frac{1}{23}$ c. $1\frac{1}{3}$ d. $1\frac{3}{5}$

Notes:

(i) Improper fractions can be converted to mixed numbers and vice versa.
(ii) The examples shown for improper fractions correspond in values to those shown for mixed numbers.

Complex Fractions a. $\frac{1/2}{7/8}$ (b) $\frac{3/4}{2/9}$

As you can see, complex fractions are "fractions over fractions".

Reducing fractions, or expressing fractions in lowest terms, is a general practice used everywhere. It makes fractions easier to read and understand.

Example: Which is easiest to understand and use?

$\frac{1}{3}$ or $\frac{17}{51}$ or $\frac{34}{102}$ They all have the same value.

In order for a number to be reduced to lowest terms, both the numerator and denominator must be divisible by the same number.

$\frac{5}{10}$

5 ← reduces to 1 when the numerator is divided by 5

10 ← reduces to 2 when the denominator is divided by 5

$\frac{3}{12}$

3 ← divided by 3 = 1

12 ← divided by 3 = 4

Note that the value of the fraction does not change.

$$\frac{5}{10} = \frac{1}{2} \qquad \frac{3}{12} = \frac{1}{4}$$

For the smaller fractions, the number used to divide is generally easy to determine.

Examples:

(a) $\frac{4}{8}$ $\frac{\text{divide by 4}}{\text{divide by 4}} = \frac{1}{2}$

(b) $\frac{3}{9}$ $\frac{\text{divide by 3}}{\text{divide by 3}} = \frac{1}{3}$

However, when the number is larger, it can be more difficult. The procedure remains the same and can be performed in multiple steps. First, find a number which will divide into both numerator and denominator. Then, inspect the resulting fraction to see if it can be further reduced.

Example: $\frac{16}{64}\left(\frac{\div 4}{\div 4}\right) = \frac{4}{16}\left(\frac{\div 4}{\div 4}\right) = \frac{1}{4}$

This example was performed in two steps. It could have been completed in one step if it had been observed that both numerator and denominator were divisible by 16.

$$\frac{16}{64}\left(\frac{\div 16}{\div 16}\right) = \frac{1}{4}$$

Some helpful hints are:

A. If both numbers are even, then they will be divisible by 2.
B. If both numbers end in 0 or 5, then they are divisible by 5.

This is often a trial-and-error procedure until proficiency is acquired. A good knowledge of both multiplication and division tables is extremely helpful.

Practice Set II-2 Reduce each of the following fractions to the lowest terms:

(a) $\frac{3}{5} =$ (b) $\frac{2}{4} =$ (c) $\frac{4}{8} =$ (d) $\frac{12}{16} =$

(e) $\frac{12}{3} =$ (f) $\frac{9}{27} =$ (g) $\frac{13}{26} =$ (h) $\frac{21}{24} =$

(i) $\frac{8}{9} =$ (j) $\frac{20}{30} =$ (k) $\frac{45}{81} =$ (l) $\frac{22}{77} =$

Improper Fractions and Mixed Numbers

An *improper fraction* is a fraction whose numerator is equal to or larger than the denominator, for example $\frac{20}{10}$ or $\frac{5}{3}$. To change improper fractions to mixed numbers, divide the denominator into the numerator for a whole number. After dividing, the remainder becomes the numerator of the fraction with the same number used as the denominator.

Example:

$\frac{7}{5}$ divide 5 into 7 which equals 1 with remainder of 2. This 2 becomes the numerator and the denominator stays at 5 $= 1\frac{2}{5}$

Here's another *example:* Convert $\frac{12}{5}$ to a mixed number.

$\frac{12}{5}$ divide 5 into 12

$$\begin{array}{r} 2 \\ 5\overline{)12} \\ -10 \\ \hline 2 \end{array}$$

determine the remainder (2)

write the mixed number $= 2\frac{2}{5}$

Examples: Reduce the following improper fractions:

(a)

$\frac{6}{5} \rightarrow$

$$\begin{array}{r} 1 \\ 5\overline{)6} \\ 5 \\ \hline 1 \end{array}$$

← remainder

$= 1\frac{1}{5}$

(b)

$$\frac{19}{6} \rightarrow 6\overline{)19} \quad 3,\; 18,\; 1 = \text{remainder} \rightarrow = 3\frac{1}{6}$$

(c)

$$\frac{18}{4} \xrightarrow{\text{divide}} 4\overline{)18} \quad 4,\; 16,\; 2 \xrightarrow{\text{rewrite}} = 4\frac{2}{4} \xrightarrow{\text{reduce to lowest terms}} = 4\frac{1}{2}$$

To change mixed numbers to improper fractions, the whole number portion is multiplied by the denominator. This new figure is then added to the numerator to become the new numerator.

add the numerator

$$2\frac{+1}{3} \rightarrow \frac{7}{3}$$

multiply

2 x 3 = 6 plus 1 is 7

denominator remains the same

Example:

$$3\frac{4}{5} = \frac{19}{5}$$

5 x 3 = 15; plus 4 is 19

denominator remains the same

Practice Set II - 3

Convert to a mixed number or an improper fraction as appropriate:

1) $\frac{10}{3} =$ 2) $\frac{17}{5} =$ 3) $\frac{25}{4} =$

4) $\frac{33}{8} =$ 5) $\frac{35}{16} =$ 6) $\frac{12}{3} =$

7) $4\frac{1}{3} =$ 8) $16\frac{1}{2} =$ 9) $1\frac{9}{10} =$

10) $5\frac{2}{7} =$ 11) $3\frac{8}{9} =$ 12) $12\frac{3}{4} =$

Practice Set II - 4

1) Reduce each fraction to lowest terms:

(a) $\frac{11}{44}$ (b) $\frac{17}{102}$ (c) $\frac{24}{25}$

(d) $\frac{12}{48}$ (e) $\frac{48}{96}$ (f) $\frac{5}{30}$

(g) $\frac{4}{32}$ (h) $\frac{3}{27}$

2) Change to improper fractions:

(a) $8\frac{7}{8}$ (b) $2\frac{13}{18}$ (c) $7\frac{5}{6}$

(d) $3\frac{5}{8}$ (e) $4\frac{11}{12}$ (f) $7\frac{5}{7}$

(g) $6\frac{8}{9}$ (h) $2\frac{5}{8}$

3) Change to mixed numbers:

(a) $\frac{51}{17}$ (b) $\frac{48}{7}$ (c) $\frac{55}{9}$

(d) $\frac{64}{9}$ (e) $\frac{85}{4}$ (f) $\frac{25}{7}$

(g) $\frac{21}{5}$ (h) $\frac{21}{4}$

Chapter 3

Multiplication and Division of Fractions

Objectives

Upon completion of this Chapter, the student must be able to do the following:

- **Multiply and Divide fractions by whole numbers.**
- **Multiply and Divide fractions by fractions.**
- **Cancel fractions.**
- **Multiply and Divide with mixed numbers and whole numbers.**
- **Multiply and Divide mixed numbers by mixed numbers.**
- **Solve problems using one or more of these operations.**

Multiplication of Fractions

Multiplication can be defined as successive addition. That is, 3 x $^1/_8$ means $\frac{1}{8}+\frac{1}{8}+\frac{1}{8}$ or $^3/_8$;

or

6 x $^2/_3$ means

$$\underbrace{\frac{2}{3}+\frac{2}{3}+\frac{2}{3}+\frac{2}{3}+\frac{2}{3}+\frac{2}{3}}_{\text{6 times}}$$

or $\frac{2}{3}+\frac{2}{3}+\frac{2}{3}+\frac{2}{3}+\frac{2}{3}+\frac{2}{3}=\frac{12}{3}=4$

Multiplication is a short cut for repeated addition and can be a time saver in the clinic. Notice in the examples given, we have been multiplying a whole number times a fraction. Fractions are typically multiplied across numerators and denominators. Since any whole number can be written with the numeral one (1) as a denominator, examine the following examples of multiplying fractions.

Example:

$4\times\frac{2}{5}$ is the same as $\frac{4}{1}\times\frac{2}{5}$ or $\frac{2}{3}\times 5=\frac{2}{3}\times\frac{5}{1}$ Why?

Multiplying:

$$\frac{4}{1}\times\frac{2}{5}=\frac{4\times 2}{1\times 5}=\frac{8}{5}=1\frac{3}{5}$$

$$\frac{2}{3}\times 5=\frac{2}{3}\times\frac{5}{1}=\frac{2\times 5}{3\times 1}=\frac{10}{3}=3\frac{1}{3}$$ which is the same as $$\frac{2}{3}+\frac{2}{3}+\frac{2}{3}+\frac{2}{3}+\frac{2}{3}=\frac{10}{3}=3\frac{1}{3}$$

Practice Set III - 1

Multiply the following fractions and whole numbers:

(a) $4\times\frac{1}{3}=$ (b) $5\times\frac{1}{4}=$ (c) $7\times\frac{1}{2}=$ (d) $18\times\frac{2}{9}=$

(e) $4\times\frac{5}{7}=$ (f) $5\times\frac{1}{2}=$ (g) $\frac{1}{3}\times 5=$ (h) $\frac{5}{6}\times 10=$

Multiplying fractions by fractions is done in the same manner. As stated previously, multiply numerator by numerator and denominator by denominator. Simplify and reduce as indicated.

Examples:

(A) $\frac{1}{3}\times\frac{1}{2}=\frac{1\times 1}{3\times 2}=\frac{1}{6}$ (B) $\frac{4}{9}\times\frac{2}{5}=\frac{4\times 2}{9\times 5}=\frac{8}{45}$

Practice Set III - 2

Multiply the following fractions. Be sure to reduce where necessary.

(a) $\frac{1}{3} \times \frac{1}{3} =$

(b) $\frac{1}{4} \times \frac{1}{4} =$

(c) $\frac{1}{3} \times \frac{1}{4} =$

(d) $\frac{2}{9} \times \frac{2}{3} =$

(e) $\frac{3}{4} \times \frac{2}{5} =$

(f) $\frac{2}{5} \times \frac{3}{5} =$

(g) $\frac{3}{4} \times \frac{5}{8} =$

(h) $\frac{7}{8} \times \frac{3}{5} =$

Now, we're going to examine a short cut that can frequently be used when multiplying fractions. Often, we can divide a numerator and a denominator by the same number and simplify the multiplication. This process is referred to as cancellation, since we "cancel" one or more of the numbers being multiplied (or some part of those numbers) which simplifies the whole process. Unfortunately, the term cancellation can confuse students; furthermore, it is not a very good description of the math concepts that allow one to "cancel".

Cancellation gets its name from the mechanics of the process as well as the effect. But, we're not really "canceling" anything - or somehow performing math magic. Rather it is based upon the principle that any number divided by itself is 1. Also, a number multiplied by 1 remains the same number. Thus,

$$\frac{5}{6} \times \frac{6}{7} = \frac{5 \times 6}{7 \times 6} = \frac{5}{7} \times 1 = \frac{5}{7}$$

(where the boxed $\frac{\times 6}{\times 6} = 1$)

As you can see, the sixes "cancel" each other; hence the term cancellation. The result is a way to "short-cut" multiplication of fractions.

$$\frac{5}{\cancel{6}} \times \frac{\cancel{6}}{7} = \frac{5}{7}$$

When can this technique be applied? Think of a bow tie. If the terms you wish to cancel are at any of the points (the darkened circles) on the bow tie, then cancellation will "work" as long as those points are connected by a line (as shown.)

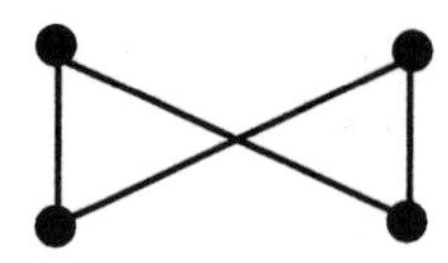

Here are some additional *examples:*

(1) $\frac{2}{\cancel{3}} \times \frac{\cancel{3}}{5} = \frac{2}{5}$

(2) $\frac{3}{\cancel{4}_1} \times \frac{\cancel{8}^2}{11} = \frac{6}{11}$ since 4 goes into 4 one time and 4 goes into 8 two times

(3) $\frac{\cancel{5}^1}{\cancel{7}_1} \times \frac{\cancel{14}^2}{\cancel{25}_5} = \frac{2}{5}$

seven into 14 twice and 5 into 25 five times

(4) $\frac{2}{3} \times \frac{2}{5} = \frac{4}{15}$ remember the bow tie? The 2's won't cancel!

(5) $\frac{{}^2\cancel{4}}{7} \times \frac{3}{\cancel{6}_3} = \frac{6}{21} = \frac{2}{7}$ 2 divides into 4 two times and into 6 three times

$\frac{{}^2\cancel{4}}{7} \times \frac{\cancel{3}^1}{\cancel{6}_{\cancel{3}_1}} = \frac{2}{7}$ same as above, but shown with the threes canceling each other

Practice Set III - 3

Multiply each of the following. Use the "cancellation" technique wherever possible.

(a) $\frac{4}{9} \times \frac{3}{5} =$

(b) $\frac{2}{5} \times \frac{3}{10} =$

(c) $\frac{2}{5} \times \frac{3}{8} =$

(d) $\frac{4}{5} \times \frac{3}{10} =$

(e) $\frac{3}{4} \times \frac{4}{5} =$

(f) $\frac{9}{10} \times \frac{4}{27} =$

(g) $\frac{2}{5} \times \frac{5}{8} =$

(h) $\frac{5}{12} \times \frac{4}{15} =$

(i) $\frac{3}{8} \times \frac{4}{9} =$

(j) $\frac{7}{8} \times \frac{2}{7} =$

(k) $\frac{2}{3} \times \frac{3}{4} \times \frac{12}{15} =$

(l) $\frac{6}{7} \times \frac{14}{15} \times \frac{5}{8} =$

In the preceding sections, you have learned how to multiply fractions by whole numbers and vice versa, how to multiply fractions by fractions and the technique of cancellation. Now, we'll learn how to multiply mixed numbers.

The only way to multiply mixed numbers is to first convert each mixed number to an improper fraction.

Recall the method for converting a mixed number to an improper fraction (from Ch 2). To change mixed numbers to improper fractions, the whole number portion is multiplied by the denominator. This new figure is then added to the numerator to become the new numerator.

add the numerator

2 x 4 plus 1 = 9

$$4\frac{+1}{2} = \frac{9}{2}$$

denominator remains the same

multiply 2 x 4

Practice Set III - 4

Change each of the following mixed numbers to improper fractions:

(a) $2\frac{1}{2} =$

(b) $3\frac{2}{3} =$

(c) $4\frac{1}{5} =$

(d) $2\frac{1}{8} =$

(e) $3\frac{5}{16} =$

To multiply a mixed number by a whole number, change the mixed number to an improper fraction and multiply; cancel if possible; and reduce to lowest terms if possible.

Example:

$$4\frac{2}{3} \times 9 = \frac{14}{3} \times 9 = \frac{14}{\cancel{3}_1} \times \frac{\cancel{9}^3}{1} = \frac{42}{1} = 42$$

Practice Set III - 5

Multiply:

(a) $5\frac{1}{3} \times 6 =$

(b) $1\frac{1}{4} \times 4 =$

(c) $8 \times 2\frac{3}{4} =$

(d) $2 \times 5\frac{3}{4} =$

(e) $6 \times 2\frac{1}{5} =$

(f) $1\frac{2}{5} \times 3 =$

When both terms are mixed numbers change both mixed numbers to improper fractions and multiply:

(g) $2\frac{2}{3} \times 3\frac{1}{2} =$

(h) $3\frac{1}{3} \times 3\frac{2}{7} =$

(i) $4\frac{1}{5} \times 2\frac{1}{3} =$

(j) $7\frac{2}{3} \times 1\frac{1}{2} =$

(k) $8\frac{1}{3} \times 6\frac{3}{4} =$

(l) $5\frac{1}{6} \times 2\frac{1}{2} =$

(m) $2\frac{3}{8} \times 3\frac{8}{16} =$

(n) $4\frac{1}{3} \times 3\frac{1}{4} =$

Applications: most of the problems you encounter in the working world are "word problems". That is, someone communicates information, verbally or written, and that information is used to solve some problem.

Practice Set III - 6

Solve the following application problems.

(a) What is the total weight of 5 dogs each weighing 8 $^{1}/_{4}$ pounds?

(b) Calculate the weight of 12 steel cages if each cage is 11 feet long and each cage weighs 2 $^{1}/_{8}$ lbs. per foot?

(c) What is the weight of 12 operating instruments, if each one weighs 1 $^{3}/_{4}$ pounds?

(d) A gallon of a certain solution requires 5 $^{7}/_{8}$ ounces of a particular chemical. How many ounces of that chemical are needed to make three gallons of solution?

Division of Fractions

Previously you learned that multiplication is a short cut to addition. The short cut to subtraction is division. Draw a line 6 inches long like the one you see here.

If you place vertical lines along this line $^1/_4$ inch apart, how many would be required? Mark it off and count them. You should have 24 vertical marks. Another way to find out the number of vertical marks needed is to divide 6 by $^1/_4$.

Example:

$6 \div \frac{1}{4} =$ The number or fraction to the right is called the divisor. In this example $^1/_4$ is the divisor.

$6 \times \frac{4}{1} =$ The next step is to invert the divisor and multiply. (The answer is 24.)

Compare the first step with the second step. How did the problem change? You should observe that the division sign was changed to a multiplication sign. Multiplication is the opposite of division; hence, the number that follows this change must be the opposite of the original number. The numerator and denominator have changed places in the divisor. When the numerator and denominator change places, we say the fraction has been *Inverted.* To invert means to turn over. A whole number like 5 when inverted becomes $^1/_5$ therefore $^1/_5$ is the *reciprocal* of 5. When dividing fractions, what we really do is multiply by the reciprocal.

Practice Set III - 7

Determine the reciprocal:

(a) 3 inverted is: (b) the reciprocal of 10 is:

(c) $^3/_5$ inverted is: (d) the reciprocal of $^5/_8$ is:

Write a rule for dividing a whole number by a fraction. Apply your rule in solving the following problem: $8 \div {}^2/_3 = ?$ If you can apply your rule to the previous problem and get 12 for an answer, you probably have a good rule. Compare your rule with the rule that follows — **To divide fractions invert the divisor and multiply.** If possible, reduce the result.

Practice Set III - 8

Solve:

(1) $5 \div {}^1/_3 =$ (2) $4 \div \frac{1}{4} =$ (3) $8 \div \frac{1}{2} =$

(4) $25 \div \frac{5}{7} =$ (5) $18 \div \frac{3}{4} =$ (6) $45 \div {}^9/_{10} =$

(7) $40 \div \frac{5}{8} =$ (8) $96 \div \frac{24}{25} =$ (9) $63 \div \frac{9}{10} =$

When dividing fractions by whole numbers, we follow the same procedure. Invert the divisor and multiply by the reciprocal.

Example: $\frac{8}{9} \div 2 =$

$\frac{8}{9} \times \frac{1}{2} =$ Notice the divisor has been inverted and the ÷ sign changed to x.

$\frac{8}{18} = \frac{4}{9}$ Reduce as indicated.

If we were to divide a fraction by a fraction, do you think the same procedure would be followed? If your answer is "Yes", you are correct. Let's try a few!

Practice Set III - 9

Divide the following fractions:

(a) $\frac{2}{3} \div \frac{4}{5} =$

(b) $\frac{5}{16} \div \frac{5}{32} =$

(c) $\frac{4}{5} \div \frac{2}{3} =$

(d) $\frac{2}{9} \div \frac{3}{4} =$

(e) $\frac{5}{12} \div \frac{3}{4} =$

(f) $\frac{9}{16} \div \frac{3}{8} =$

(g) $\frac{7}{8} \div \frac{5}{12} =$

(h) $\frac{3}{16} \div \frac{9}{32} =$

Application:

(i) A cafe owner used a $^{3}/_{4}$ pound can of pepper to fill the pepper shakers. Each shaker can hold $^{1}/_{64}$ pound of pepper. In this way, how many shakers would she fill from the $^{3}/_{4}$ pound can?

When multiplying mixed numbers we first had to change any mixed numbers to improper fractions. The same procedure must be followed when dividing mixed numbers. To divide fractions involving mixed numbers change the mixed number to an improper fraction; invert the divisor, multiply, cancel where possible.

Example 1:

$3\frac{1}{2} \div 4$ change the mixed number to an improper fraction

$\frac{7}{2} \div 4$ change to multiplication and use the reciprocal of the divisor

$\frac{7}{2} \times \frac{1}{4} = \frac{7}{8}$

Example 2 :

$5\frac{1}{3} \div 2\frac{2}{3}$ change mixed numbers to improper fractions

$\frac{16}{3} \div \frac{8}{3}$ invert the divisor and multiply

$\frac{16}{3} \times \frac{3}{8}$

$\frac{\overset{2}{\cancel{16}}}{\underset{1}{\cancel{3}}} \times \frac{\overset{1}{\cancel{3}}}{\underset{1}{\cancel{8}}} = \frac{2}{1} = 2$ multiply and simplify

Note the use of cancellation techniques.

Practice Set III - 10

Divide:

(a) $6\frac{2}{3} \div \frac{1}{4} =$

(b) $5\frac{3}{5} \div 7 =$

(c) $4\frac{1}{3} \div 10 =$

(d) $\frac{3}{5} \div \frac{9}{10} =$

(e) $\frac{5}{8} \div 2\frac{1}{2} =$

(f) $4\frac{1}{5} \div 1\frac{3}{4} =$

(g) $30 \div 1\frac{2}{3} =$

(h) $17\frac{1}{2} \div 3\frac{1}{2} =$

(i) $6\frac{2}{5} \div 5\frac{1}{3} =$

(j) $85 \div 4\frac{1}{4} =$

Practice Set III - 11

Review. Perform the indicated operation and simplify.

(a) $\frac{7}{8} \times \frac{8}{9} =$

(b) $1\frac{2}{3} \times \frac{3}{10} =$

(c) $\frac{4}{5} \times \frac{1}{2} =$

(d) $2 \times \frac{5}{8} \times 1\frac{3}{4} =$

(e) $\frac{6}{8} \times \frac{2}{3} =$

(f) $3\frac{1}{2} \times \frac{12}{8} \times 1\frac{1}{2} =$

(g) $\frac{17}{51} \times \frac{1}{2} =$

(h) $\frac{3}{3} \times \frac{2}{2} \times \frac{5}{5} =$

(i) $\frac{9}{10} \times \frac{5}{3} =$

(j) $\frac{1}{2} \div \frac{1}{4} =$

(k) $\frac{9}{10} \times 1\frac{2}{3} =$

(l) $\frac{1}{6} \div \frac{1}{8} =$

(m) $1\frac{2}{3} \times 3\frac{1}{5} =$

(n) $\frac{1}{3} \div \frac{2}{7} =$

(o) $24 \times \frac{1}{2} =$

(p) $1\frac{2}{5} \div \frac{3}{10} =$

(q) $24 \times \frac{1}{3} =$

(r) $2\frac{6}{10} \div \frac{10}{14} =$

(s) $24 \times \frac{2}{3} =$

(t) $8\frac{8}{10} \div \frac{11}{5} =$

(u) $24 \times \frac{3}{3} =$

(v)
$$2\frac{3}{4} \div \frac{11}{16} =$$

(w)
$$\frac{3}{4} \times \frac{2}{3} \times \frac{1}{2} =$$

(x)
$$3\frac{4}{5} \div 6\frac{7}{8} =$$

(y)
$$1\frac{2}{3} \div 4\frac{5}{6} =$$

(z)
$$9 \div \frac{1}{3} =$$

(aa)
$$4 \div \frac{1}{2} =$$

(bb)
$$\frac{1}{2} \div \frac{1}{4} =$$

(cc)
$$\frac{2}{5} \div 1\frac{1}{4} =$$

(dd)
$$\frac{8}{11} \div \frac{16}{22} =$$

(ee)
$$4\frac{3}{5} \div \frac{23}{30} =$$

(ff)
$$\frac{3}{3} \div \frac{2}{2} =$$

(gg)
$$2\frac{1}{2} \div 2\frac{1}{2} =$$

Chapter 4

Addition and Subtraction of Fractions

Objectives

Upon completion of this Chapter, the student must be able to do the following:

- **Add and Subtract proper fractions with common denominator.**
- **Determine common denominators for fractions.**
- **Add and Subtract fractions with unlike denominators.**
- **Add and Subtract mixed numbers.**
- **Add and Subtract improper fractions.**

Addition of Fractions

Adding fractions with common denominators

To add or subtract fractions, a common denominator is required. To add fractions with a common denominator, add the numerators and write this sum over the common denominator.

Example:

add the numerators

$$\frac{1}{5}+\frac{2}{5}=\frac{1+2}{5}=\frac{3}{5}$$

retain the common denominator

The numerators 1 and 2 are added and their sum (3) is written over the common denominator (5). Reduce any fraction, if possible; and convert any improper fraction to a mixed number.

Practice Set IV - 1

Add the following fractions. Be sure to reduce where necessary:

(a) $\frac{3}{8}+\frac{4}{8}=$ (b) $\frac{9}{16}+\frac{1}{16}=$ (c) $\frac{3}{5}+\frac{1}{5}=$

(d) $\frac{7}{16} + \frac{5}{16}$

(e) $\frac{1}{7} + \frac{2}{7}$

(f) $\frac{5}{8} + \frac{1}{8} + \frac{3}{8}$

(g) $\frac{2}{16} + \frac{11}{16} + \frac{7}{16}$

Adding Fractions with Different Denominators

Fractions cannot be added unless they have a common denominator. Fractions have a common denominator when all their denominators are the same, as $\frac{5}{8}$, $\frac{7}{8}$, and $\frac{3}{8}$.

Example:

$\frac{2}{3}+\frac{3}{4}+\frac{1}{2}=?$ Fractions without common denominators.

When the denominators are not the same, make them the same. How? First determine a common denominator, preferably, the **LCD** (*least common denominator*). That is, find the smallest number into which all the given denominators will divide evenly. In this example, the lowest number into which all the denominators (3, 4, and 2) will evenly divide is 12. This will be the least common denominator.

The next step is to adjust the denominator in each fraction to a common denominator.

$$\frac{2}{3} \times \frac{}{4} = \frac{}{12}$$

$$\frac{3}{4} \times \frac{}{3} = \frac{}{12}$$

$$\frac{1}{2} \times \frac{}{6} = \frac{}{12}$$

by multiplying each denominator by a different number, we achieve the common denominator in each case

Then adjust the numerators in a similar fashion. Recall that any number multiplied by 1 is the same number; its value doesn't change. Furthermore, any fraction which has the same numerator and denominator is equal to 1. Since each denominator was multiplied by a different number in order to reach 12, multiply the numerators by that same number in each case.

$$\frac{2}{3} \times \frac{4}{4} = \frac{8}{12}$$

$$\frac{3}{4} \times \frac{3}{3} = \frac{9}{12}$$

$$\frac{1}{2} \times \frac{6}{6} = \frac{6}{12}$$

multiplying each fraction by the same number with which we achieved the denominator, adjusts the numerator.

Now we have a common denominator and the fractions can be added.

$$\frac{2}{3} \times \frac{4}{4} = \frac{8}{12}$$

$$\frac{3}{4} \times \frac{3}{3} = \frac{9}{12}$$

$$+ \frac{1}{2} \times \frac{6}{6} = \frac{6}{12}$$

$$\frac{23}{12}$$

Reduce to simplest form $\frac{23}{12} = 1\frac{11}{12}$

Practice Set IV - 2

Add the fractions; remember to find the LCD first; and reduce to simplest form where possible:

(a) $\frac{1}{12} + \frac{1}{4}$ (b) $\frac{1}{6} + \frac{1}{3}$ (c) $\frac{1}{2} + \frac{1}{6}$

(d) $\frac{1}{4} + \frac{1}{2}$

(e) $\frac{2}{12} + \frac{1}{4}$

(f) $\frac{3}{8} + \frac{1}{4}$

(g)
$\frac{1}{8}$
$\frac{1}{2}$

(h)
$\frac{3}{6}$
$\frac{1}{3}$

(i)
$\frac{1}{8}$
$\frac{1}{4}$

(j)
$\frac{2}{6}$
$\frac{1}{2}$

(k) $\frac{1}{7}+\frac{1}{2}$

(l)
$\frac{3}{8}$
$\frac{3}{4}$

(m)
$\frac{1}{16}$
$\frac{1}{24}$
$\frac{3}{48}$
$\frac{1}{6}$

(n)
$\frac{1}{4}$
$\frac{3}{8}$
$\frac{3}{4}$
$\frac{5}{6}$

(o)
$\frac{5}{6}$
$\frac{1}{8}$
$\frac{2}{3}$

(p)
$\frac{3}{5}$
$\frac{4}{6}$
$\frac{7}{8}$

Adding Mixed Numbers

A mixed number is a number composed of a whole number and a fraction taken together, such as $3\frac{2}{5}$ or $1\frac{2}{3}$. To add mixed numbers — add the whole numbers and the fractions separately and combine the results. Simplify and reduce as needed.

Example:

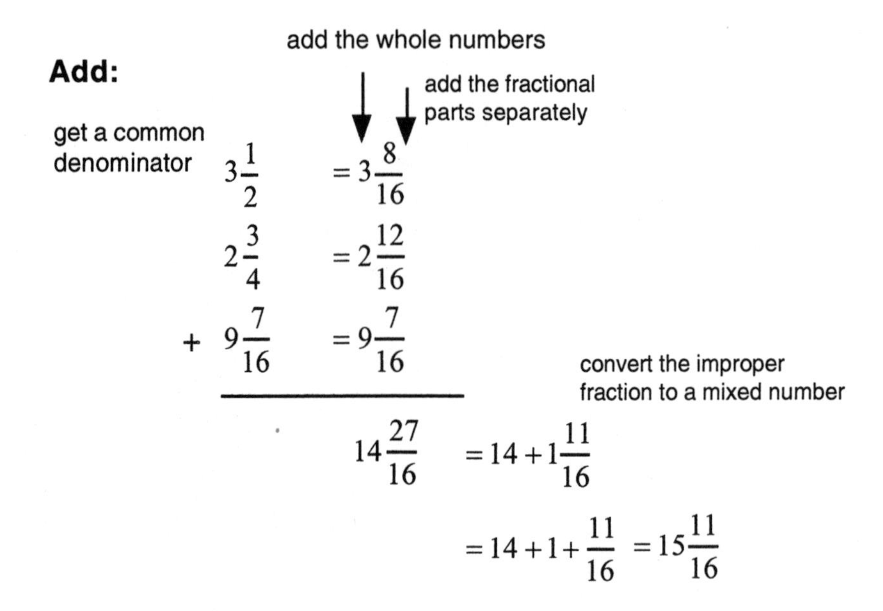

In this example (above), the fractions were changed to 16ths (for a common denominator) and added for a sum of $\frac{27}{16}$, which simplifies to $1\frac{11}{16}$. The sum of the whole numbers was 14. Combining these results yields the solution $15\frac{11}{16}$.

Another procedure for adding mixed numbers involves changing all the mixed numbers to improper fractions before adding. That procedure, while correct, tends to involve more steps thus increasing the possibility for error. If you know how to do this procedure, and are comfortable with doing it, then you are welcome to do so. In math, there are often several ways to a solution. Rarely, though, is there only one "right" way. Any method that is mathematically sound and achieves the desired result is acceptable.

Practice Set IV - 3

Add:

(a)
$$\begin{array}{r} 5\frac{1}{3} \\ +\ 8\frac{1}{12} \\ \hline \end{array}$$

(b)
$$\begin{array}{r} 4\frac{3}{5} \\ +\ 6\frac{1}{10} \\ \hline \end{array}$$

(c)
$$\begin{array}{r} 7\frac{2}{4} \\ +\ 12\frac{1}{8} \\ \hline \end{array}$$

(d)
$$\begin{array}{r} 8\frac{3}{10} \\ +\ 9\frac{2}{5} \\ \hline \end{array}$$

(e)
$$\begin{array}{r} 8\frac{1}{2} \\ +\ 7\frac{1}{4} \\ \hline \end{array}$$

(f)
$$\begin{array}{r} 14\frac{1}{6} \\ +\ 6\frac{1}{3} \\ \hline \end{array}$$

(g)
$$\begin{array}{r} 15\frac{1}{10} \\ +\ 7\frac{1}{2} \\ \hline \end{array}$$

(h)
$$\begin{array}{r} 9\frac{3}{8} \\ +\ 8\frac{1}{4} \\ \hline \end{array}$$

(i)
$$\begin{array}{r} 6\frac{6}{16} \\ +\ 7\frac{1}{8} \\ \hline \end{array}$$

(j)
$$\begin{array}{r} 12\frac{1}{4} \\ +\ 7\frac{1}{12} \\ \hline \end{array}$$

(k)
$$\begin{array}{r} 6\frac{7}{10} \\ +\ 8\frac{4}{5} \\ \hline \end{array}$$

(l)
$$\begin{array}{r} 4\frac{3}{5} \\ +\ 7\frac{11}{15} \\ \hline \end{array}$$

(m)
$$\begin{array}{r} 9\frac{5}{6} \\ +\ 6\frac{2}{3} \\ \hline \end{array}$$

(n)
$$\begin{array}{r} 7\frac{1}{2} \\ +\ 9\frac{3}{8} \\ \hline \end{array}$$

(o)
$$\begin{array}{r} 3\frac{1}{9} \\ +\ 5\frac{2}{3} \\ \hline \end{array}$$

Adding Improper Fractions

Improper fractions can be added in two ways: (1) Convert the improper fraction(s) to mixed numbers and add as previously shown; or (2) Determine the common denominator, add the fractions and then convert the answer to a mixed number.

Example:

$$\begin{array}{rl} \frac{3}{2} & = \frac{9}{6} \\ \frac{5}{3} & = \frac{10}{6} \\ +\frac{7}{6} & = \frac{7}{6} \\ \hline & \frac{26}{6} = 4\frac{2}{6} = 4\frac{1}{3} \end{array}$$

Determine LCD, adjust numerators and add

Convert to mixed number and reduce to lowest terms

Practice Set IV - 4

Add the following:

(a) $\frac{17}{16}$ $\frac{9}{8}$ $+\frac{3}{2}$

(b) $\frac{3}{2}$ $\frac{5}{4}$ $+\frac{11}{8}$

(c) $\frac{7}{5}$ $\frac{9}{4}$ $+\frac{12}{10}$

(d) $\frac{27}{9}$ $\frac{24}{8}$ $+\frac{3}{2}$

Combinations of mixed numbers, whole numbers, and fractions — common and improper — are combined similarly.

Practice Set IV - 5

Add the following:

(a) $1\frac{3}{4}$ $\frac{5}{3}$ $+\frac{1}{2}$

(b) $4\frac{3}{5}$ $6\frac{3}{8}$ $+\frac{23}{20}$

(c) $2\frac{1}{2}$ $3\frac{3}{2}$ $+2\frac{2}{3}$

(d) $4\frac{3}{16}$ $3\frac{2}{8}$ $2\frac{1}{4}$ $+1\frac{1}{2}$

Subtraction of Fractions

Subtracting fractions is very similar to adding fractions except now the arithmetic operation is subtraction. Nearly everything else you've learned about adding fractions applies to subtracting them as well.

To subtract proper fractions with like denominators, subtract the numerators and place the result over the common denominator. Remember to reduce or simplify if possible.

Example:

Vertically

$$\begin{array}{r} \frac{9}{16} \\ -\frac{7}{16} \\ \hline \frac{2}{16} = \frac{1}{8} \end{array}$$

Or horizontally

$$\frac{9}{16} - \frac{7}{16} = \frac{9-7}{16} = \frac{2}{16} = \frac{1}{8}$$

Practice Set IV - 6

Subtract the following fractions with like denominators.

(a) $\begin{array}{r} \frac{2}{3} \\ -\frac{1}{3} \\ \hline \end{array}$ (b) $\begin{array}{r} \frac{5}{6} \\ -\frac{4}{6} \\ \hline \end{array}$ (c) $\begin{array}{r} \frac{8}{11} \\ -\frac{1}{11} \\ \hline \end{array}$ (d) $\begin{array}{r} \frac{13}{16} \\ -\frac{5}{16} \\ \hline \end{array}$

When subtracting fractions with unlike denominators, first determine a common denominator, then adjust the numerators as needed and subtract. This is exactly as you have done when adding fractions.

Example:

$$\begin{array}{rr} \frac{5}{8} & = \frac{5}{8} \\ -\frac{1}{4} & = -\frac{2}{8} \\ \hline & \frac{3}{8} \end{array}$$

Practice Set IV - 7

Subtract:

(a) $\frac{3}{4} - \frac{3}{8}$

(b) $\frac{5}{8} - \frac{1}{2}$

(c) $\frac{1}{3} - \frac{1}{6}$

(d) $\frac{1}{2} - \frac{3}{16}$

(e) $\frac{15}{32} - \frac{1}{4}$

(f) $\frac{1}{16} - \frac{1}{32}$

(g) $\frac{17}{20} - \frac{1}{2}$

(h) $\frac{9}{15} - \frac{1}{3}$

(i) $\frac{11}{4} - \frac{1}{2}$

(j) $\frac{15}{8} - \frac{1}{4}$

(k) $\frac{11}{10} - \frac{1}{2}$

(l) $\frac{16}{12} - \frac{1}{2}$

(m) $\frac{12}{10} - \frac{1}{5}$

(n) $\frac{12}{9} - \frac{1}{3}$

Subtracting Mixed Numbers

Subtract mixed numbers just as you added them — subtract the fractions, then subtract the whole numbers.

Example:

$$11\frac{5}{6} = 11\frac{10}{12}$$

$$-3\frac{3}{4} = -3\frac{9}{12}$$

$$8\frac{1}{12}$$

Determine the LCD and convert the fractions

$$\frac{10}{12} - \frac{9}{12} = \frac{1}{12}$$

and

$$11 - 3 = 8$$

Practice Set IV - 8

Subtract these mixed numbers. Be sure to reduce to lowest terms where possible.

(a) $7\frac{5}{8} - 4\frac{1}{4}$

(b) $9\frac{5}{8} - 5\frac{1}{2}$

(c) $8\frac{3}{4} - 5\frac{5}{8}$

(d) $15\frac{3}{4} - 11\frac{1}{2}$

(e) $13\frac{11}{18} - 12\frac{4}{9}$

(f) $10\frac{2}{5} - 3\frac{1}{4}$

(g) $9\frac{3}{4} - \frac{2}{3}$

(h) $62\frac{7}{10} - 50\frac{7}{20}$

(i) $6\frac{2}{3} - 3\frac{1}{5}$

(j) $14\frac{1}{2} - 2\frac{1}{4}$

Subtracting mixed numbers where the subtrahend is a larger fraction

Example:

$2\frac{1}{4}$ minuend - the number from which another is being subtracted

$-\frac{3}{4}$ Subtrahend - the number which is subtracted

Note that we wish to subtract $\frac{3}{4}$ from $\frac{1}{4}$. But $\frac{3}{4}$ is larger than $\frac{1}{4}$.

This procedure can only be completed by "borrowing". Borrow a whole number (1), change it into a fraction and add it to the minuend; then subtract.

Example:

$^{1}\not{2}\frac{1}{4}$ borrow 1(whole unit) from the 2

$-\frac{3}{4}$

$^{1}\not{2}\frac{\not{1}^{5}}{4}$ add the numerator and denominator together creating a new numerator

$-\frac{3}{4}$

$1\frac{5}{4}$ this is the new Minuend

$-\frac{3}{4}$

$1\frac{2}{4} = 1\frac{1}{2}$ subtract and reduce

Here is the same problem shown another way:

Borrow one from the two, convert to a fraction ($1 = \frac{4}{4}$), then subtract. Reduce if possible.

$$\begin{array}{r} 2\frac{1}{4} \\ -\frac{3}{4} \\ \hline \end{array} = \begin{array}{r} 1 + 1\frac{1}{4} \\ -\frac{3}{4} \\ \hline \end{array} = \begin{array}{r} 1 + \frac{4}{4} + \frac{1}{4} \\ -\frac{3}{4} \\ \hline \end{array} = \begin{array}{r} 1\frac{5}{4} \\ -\frac{3}{4} \\ \hline 1\frac{2}{4} = 1\frac{1}{2} \end{array}$$

In practical terms, all you have to remember is to add the numerator and denominator (as in the first example) after you borrow. This works (as shown in detail in the second example) because any number over itself (that is, any time the numerator and denominator are the same) is equal to one. So if you borrow one whole number it will equal the same number of parts in which the fraction is represented.

If unlike denominators are represented, first determine the common denominator, then borrow and subtract. Here's an *example* ...

$$\begin{array}{r} 3\frac{1}{5} \\ -1\frac{2}{3} \\ \hline \end{array} \quad \text{determine the LCD} \quad \begin{array}{r} 3\frac{3}{15} \\ -1\frac{10}{15} \\ \hline \end{array} \quad \text{borrow} \quad \begin{array}{r} 2\not{3}\frac{\not{3}\,18}{15} \\ -1\frac{10}{15} \\ \hline \end{array} \quad \text{Add the numerator and denominator} \quad \begin{array}{r} 2\frac{18}{15} \\ -1\frac{10}{15} \\ \hline 1\frac{8}{15} \end{array} \quad \text{Subtract}$$

Practice Set IV - 9

Subtract the following mixed numbers:

(a) $\begin{array}{r} 3\frac{2}{5} \\ -\ 2\frac{2}{3} \\ \hline \end{array}$ (b) $\begin{array}{r} 4\frac{3}{4} \\ -\ 1\frac{7}{8} \\ \hline \end{array}$ (c) $\begin{array}{r} 2\frac{1}{3} \\ -\frac{5}{6} \\ \hline \end{array}$ (d) $\begin{array}{r} 1\frac{3}{4} \\ -\frac{7}{8} \\ \hline \end{array}$ (e) $\begin{array}{r} 2\frac{3}{11} \\ -\frac{7}{22} \\ \hline \end{array}$

(f) $\begin{array}{r} 16 \\ -\frac{1}{2} \\ \hline \end{array}$ (g) $\begin{array}{r} 8 \\ -\frac{4}{5} \\ \hline \end{array}$ (h) $\begin{array}{r} 1\frac{4}{9} \\ -\frac{13}{18} \\ \hline \end{array}$ (i) $\begin{array}{r} 1\frac{9}{20} \\ -\frac{4}{5} \\ \hline \end{array}$ (j) $\begin{array}{r} 9 \\ -\frac{9}{18} \\ \hline \end{array}$

Subtracting Improper Fractions

Except for the operation (subtraction), the techniques for subtracting are the same as for addition of improper fractions.

Examples:

(1) $\begin{array}{r} \frac{11}{8} \\ -\ \frac{9}{8} \\ \hline \frac{2}{8} = \frac{1}{4} \end{array}$

(2) $\begin{array}{r} \frac{16}{4} = \frac{32}{8} \\ -\ \frac{3}{8} = \frac{3}{8} \\ \hline \frac{29}{8} = 3\frac{5}{8} \end{array}$ determine the LCD; convert to mixed number; reduce if necessary

Practice Set IV - 10

Subtract the following:

(a) $\dfrac{11}{9} - \dfrac{10}{9}$

(b) $\dfrac{11}{9} - \dfrac{4}{18}$

(c) $\dfrac{5}{4} - \dfrac{6}{5}$

(d) $\dfrac{6}{5} - \dfrac{7}{6}$

(e) $\dfrac{51}{18} - \dfrac{1}{9}$

Practice Set IV - Chapter Review

Solve each of the following:

(a) $\dfrac{11}{17}+\dfrac{8}{34}$

(b) $1\dfrac{11}{17}-\dfrac{8}{34}$

(c) $\dfrac{1}{8}+\dfrac{1}{16}+\dfrac{3}{2}$

(d) $4\dfrac{1}{9}+6\dfrac{11}{18}+9\dfrac{1}{3}$

(e) $\dfrac{6}{8}-\dfrac{3}{5}$

(f) $4\dfrac{1}{8}-1\dfrac{5}{7}$

(g) $1\dfrac{1}{2}+2\dfrac{2}{3}+3\dfrac{3}{4}+4\dfrac{4}{5}$

(h) $4\dfrac{3}{4}-3\dfrac{4}{5}$

(i) $4\dfrac{7}{8}-2\dfrac{8}{9}$

(j) $6\frac{2}{3}-\frac{3}{4}$

(k) $1\frac{16}{17}-\frac{32}{34}$

(l) $\frac{7}{8}-\frac{2}{3}$

(m) $14\frac{5}{12}-6\frac{9}{10}$

(n) $8\frac{3}{5}-\frac{7}{10}$

(o) $1\frac{5}{24}-\frac{1}{4}$

(p) $\frac{2}{3}-\frac{2}{6}$

(q) $1\frac{4}{9}-\frac{4}{18}$

(r) $4\frac{2}{6}-\frac{4}{9}$

(s) $4\frac{2}{7}-\frac{1}{2}$

(t) $8-\frac{4}{9}$

(u) $18\frac{1}{24}-1\frac{7}{8}$

(v) $\frac{1}{3}-\frac{1}{8}$

(w) $\frac{4}{16}-\frac{1}{4}$

(x) $7\frac{1}{4}-\frac{2}{3}$

Chapter 5

Decimal Fractions

Part I

Objectives

Upon completion, the student must be able to do the following:

- **Add and Subtract decimal fractions.**
- **Express a common fraction as a decimal fraction.**
- **Convert decimal fractions to common fractions.**

In the first few chapters we studied the four operations of common fractions. Now we study a different fraction that is very important and has everyday applications in the clinic and at the lab. The new fraction to be studied in this section is the decimal fraction. A *decimal fraction* may be considered a common fraction whose denominator is 10 or some power of 10, such as 100 (10^2); 1,000 (10^3) and so on.

Examples: $\frac{3}{10}$ can be written .3 or 0.3

$\frac{21}{100}$ can be written .21 or 0.21

$\frac{297}{1000}$ can be written .297

321 .234567

All numbers to the left of the decimal point are *whole numbers.*

One place to the right of the decimal point is ten*ths*; two places to the right of the decimal point is hundred*ths*, three places thousand*ths*, the fourth decimal place indicates ten-thousand*ths* and the fifth decimal place to the right of the decimal is the hundred-thousand*ths* place. When reading the decimal point, we say "and".

Example: 2.57 is read two *and* fifty-seven hundredths

An alternate method involves the words "decimal" or "point" and read the numerals as:

2.57 read as two *point* five seven or two *decimal* fifty-seven

When writing (or reading) decimals of small values, less than one for example, zeros are placed between the decimal point and the number in the decimal (if necessary).

Examples:

seven hundredths is written .07
nine thousandths .009

Practice Set V - 1

Write the following as decimal fractions [as shown in (a)]:

(a) nine tenths = .9

(b) three tenths =

(c) twenty-five hundredths =

(d) nine ten-thousandths =

(e) twelve thousandths =

(f) twenty-two thousandths of an inch =

(g) five tenths feet =

(h) thirty-two thousandths =

Remember, decimals are really fractions, or parts, of a whole. We use these instead of common fractions because decimal fractions are easier since they're based on powers of ten. We can easily change common fractions to decimal fractions by dividing the numerator by the denominator.

Example: Change $\frac{5}{8}$ to a decimal fraction.

$$8\overline{)5.000}^{\;.625}$$

Divide 5 by 8. Since 8 does not evenly divide into 5, we place the decimal point after the 5 (in the dividend), and immediately above that in the answer (the quotient). Add zeros to the dividend and complete the division.

To convert a mixed number to a decimal, keep the whole number and convert the fractional part to a decimal as in the previous example.

$$1\frac{3}{4} = 1.75 \qquad \text{since} \quad 4\overline{)3.00}^{\,.75}$$

Practice Set V - 2

Change the following common fractions to decimal fractions.

(a) $\frac{11}{64}$ (b) $\frac{3}{32}$ (c) $\frac{5}{8}$ (d) $\frac{5}{16}$ (e) $\frac{1}{4}$

(f) $\frac{1}{8}$ (g) $\frac{5}{64}$ (h) $\frac{1}{2}$ (i) $1\frac{3}{8}$ (j) $1\frac{7}{16}$

(k) $\frac{3}{4}$ (l) $\frac{7}{8}$ (m) $2\frac{5}{8}$ (n) $\frac{3}{80}$ (o) $1\frac{9}{64}$

To change decimal fractions to common fractions:

Example: change .45 to a common fraction.

$$.45 = \frac{45}{100} = \frac{9}{20} \text{ (reduced)}$$

decimal fraction (.45) — common fractions ($\frac{45}{100}$, $\frac{9}{20}$)

In other words, change the decimal fraction to its equivalent common fraction; reduce to lowest terms if possible.

Tip: count the decimal places and that indicates the number of zeros for the denominator.

Examples: (a) $0.456 = \frac{456}{1000}$

three decimal places, thus three zeros

(b) $0.0076 = \frac{76}{10{,}000}$

four decimal places, thus four zeros

Practice Set V - 3

Change each of the following to common fractions and reduce to lowest terms.

(a) .06 (b) .250 (c) .495 (d) .33

(e) .630 (f) .009 (g) .3 (h) .3755 (i) 1.188

Addition of Decimals

You already know how to add dollars and cents. Add decimals the same way! The key to remember is to align the decimal points in a column; add just as you would for whole numbers, placing the decimal point in the answer directly below the column of decimal points.

Example: Add: 6.25 + 21.021 + 873.0725 + 647

```
   6.25
  21.021
 873.0725
 647.      <——  a common error involves "forgetting" that the decimal in a
 ________       whole number belongs at the right end of that number
```

Some students like to even the columns using zeros in those numbers with fewer places so everything "lines up". Like this:

```
   6.2500
  21.0210
 873.0725
 647.0000
1547.3435
_________
```

Practice Set V - 4

Add the following :

(a) 0.008, 20, 0.6, 4.5

(b) 0.03, 0.3, 4.12, 30

(c) 10, 0.0615, 1.2

(d) 52.2, 0.06, 0.0008, 2000

(e) 0.005, 2.5, 1.1

(f) 0.006, 5, 0.32, 0.08

(g) 0.05, 10.256, 12.2

(h) 0.09, 10, 4.8, 1000

(i) 0.05, 0.006, 0.032, 0.0003

(j) 2.5, 1.98, 100, 0.8

(k) 1.2, 1.5, 0.03, 15

(l) 0.15, 0.4, 0.048, 6

(m) 0.8, 1.5, 0.5

(n) 0.64, 8, 0.06, 0.3

Subtraction of Decimals

Subtraction of decimals in done in a similar manner. Align the decimal points, subtract, place the decimal in the answer directly in the same column as the aligned decimals. Again, you may add zeros so that all numbers align.

Example: subtract 15.275 from 32.63

$$\begin{array}{r} 32.63 \\ -15.275 \\ \hline \end{array} \quad \text{or} \quad \begin{array}{r} 32.630 \\ -15.275 \\ \hline 17.355 \end{array}$$

Practice Set V - 5

Subtract :

(a) 92.12 minus .37

(b) 1,000 minus 810.77

(c) 11,246.51 minus 247.59

(d) 53.36 minus 43.65

(e) .0257 from 9.3126

(f) 4.695 from 7.342

(g) .079 from .1032

(h) .65832 from 1

Decimal Fractions

Part II

Objectives

Upon completion, the student must be able to do the following:

- **Multiply with decimals.**
- **Divide with decimals.**
- **Round answers to desired number of places.**

Multiplication of Decimals

In the previous section you learned how to add and subtract with decimals. In this section, we learn how to multiply and divide with decimals.

When multiplying numbers, the result, or answer, is called the product.

Examples: $5 \times 12 = 60$ (the product is 60)

$\frac{1}{2} \times \frac{2}{3} = \frac{2}{6} = \frac{1}{3}$ (product is 1/3)

$0.3 \times 0.5 = 0.15$ (product is 0.15)

Note in the examples above, it doesn't matter if the numbers are whole numbers, common fractions, or decimal fractions - the answer is called the product in each case of multiplication.

When multiplying decimals, proceed as in multiplying whole numbers. The process is the same. The only change is placing the decimal point in the proper position in the resultant product. Count the number of decimal places in each of the numbers multiplied.

Example:

$$\begin{array}{r} .12 \\ \times \underline{\quad 5} \end{array}$$

In the numbers above, 5 and .12, How many decimal places are there? ____________

Your answer should have two decimal places. In the product start at the rightmost digit and count two decimal places to the left:

$$\begin{array}{r} .12 \\ \times\underline{5} \\ .60 \end{array}$$ <-- two decimal places in the product!

Practice Set V - 6

Determine the placement of the decimal point for each of the product shown:

(a)	(b)	(c)	(d)	(e)
$\begin{array}{r} .35 \\ \times\underline{\quad 4} \\ 140 \end{array}$	$\begin{array}{r} 94 \\ \underline{\times .4} \\ 376 \end{array}$	$\begin{array}{r} .707 \\ \times\underline{\quad .2} \\ 1414 \end{array}$	$\begin{array}{r} 1.6 \\ \times\underline{\quad 40} \\ 640 \end{array}$	$\begin{array}{r} .0638 \\ \underline{\times .78} \\ 49764 \end{array}$

Note: in (e) the sum of the decimal points to be counted off is six. Yet the product has only five digits. In these cases, add one or more zeros to the ***left*** of the product in order to have the required number of decimal places. The answer for (e) should be: .049764

Practice Set V - 7

Multiply. Place the decimal point in the correct position in the product.

(a) $17.5 \times 6 =$

(b) $168 \times 0.321 =$

(c) $4.8 \times .067 =$

(d) $0.56 \times 0.83 =$

(e) $63 \times 37.91 =$

(f) $0.72 \times 0.095 =$

(g)
Multiply 0.2279 by 0.029

(h)
Multiply 6.85 by 81.2

(i)
306.693×2.61

(j)
Find the product of 18.35 and 0.065

(k)
29 hours of work at $5.12 per hour is ?

(l)
Find the cost of 212 bushels of corn at $3.08 per bushel.

(m)
98 bushels of feed at $5.88 a bushel = ?

(n)
How much is 32 quarts of milk at $1.19 a quart?

(o)
18 dozen eggs at $1.55 per dozen is ?

In the lab, you will often need to multiply by 10 or 100 or one thousand. These all represent multiples of ten. There is a short cut to multiplying by multiples of ten. For example, multiply 2.4 by 10, 100, and 1000.

$$2.4 \times 10 = 24$$
$$2.4 \times 100 = 240.0$$
$$2.4 \times 1000 = 2400.0$$

Notice that when 2.4 is multiplied by 10, How does the decimal place change in the product?

When multiplying by ten, the decimal is moved to the right one place in the product. When multiplying by 1,000 the decimal point is moved three places to the right in the product. Can you make a rule for use when multiplying by powers of ten?

____

____

Practice Set V - 8

Multiply the following. Try using the rule you just formulated.

(a) 3.6×10

(b) 5.4×1000

(c) $.47 \times 100$

(d) 9.61×100

(e) 2.45×1000

(f) 7.1×10

Division of Decimals

Next we learn how to divide using decimals. Recall that in multiplication the answer, or result is called the product. In division, the answer is called the quotient. The number that is being divided is called the dividend; and the number with which the dividend is divided is called the divisor.

Example:

$$divisor\overline{)dividend}^{\;quotient}$$

divisor → $6\overline{)42}$ ← dividend, with 7 ← quotient above

Suppose we wanted to divide a whole number by some decimal number. Such as: $.16\overline{)32}$

The divisor is 0.16 and the dividend is 32. With division, the divisor must always be made into a whole number by moving the decimal place to the right. In this case, the decimal point is moved two places to the right. To allow this procedure, we must also then move the decimal place of the dividend two places to the right as well. Finally, place the decimal point in the quotient, the answer, directly above the new position in the dividend. Like this

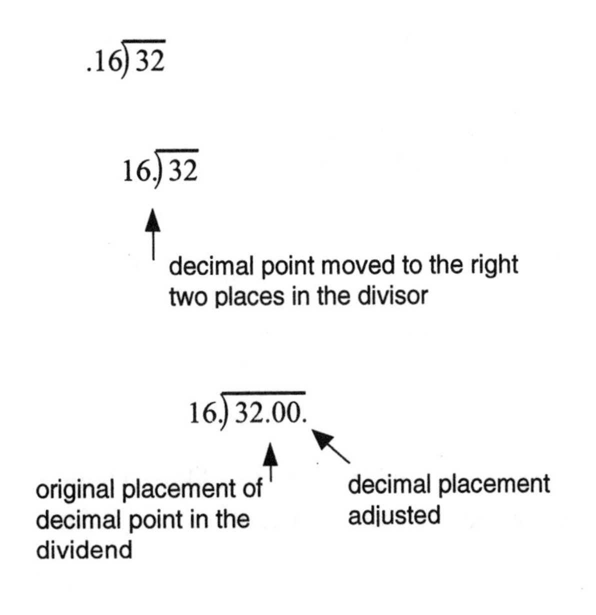

Finally, do the division: $\begin{array}{r} 200. \\ 16.\overline{)3200.} \end{array}$

Practice Set V - 9

Divide :

(a) $1.2\overline{)36}$

(b) $1.3\overline{)650}$

(c) $.5\overline{)75}$

(d) $.08\overline{)64}$

(e) $.9\overline{)72}$

(f) $.25\overline{)200}$

From (f), here is another look at that problem.

$$.25\overline{)200} = 200 \div .25$$

$$= 200 \div \frac{1}{4} \quad \text{since } 0.25 = \frac{1}{4}$$

$$= 200 \times \frac{4}{1} \quad \text{as learned when dividing fractions}$$

$$= 800$$

To divide a decimal by a whole number, divide as you would for whole numbers and place the decimal point in the quotient directly above the decimal point in the dividend.

Examples:

$$16\overline{)6.4}\ \text{quotient } .4 \qquad 22\overline{).88}\ \text{quotient } .04 \qquad 13\overline{)26.}\ \text{quotient } 2.$$

Practice Set V - 10

Divide :

(a) $25\overline{)6.50}$ (b) $44\overline{)9.24}$ (c) $16\overline{).922}$

(d) $14\overline{).42}$ (e) $12\overline{)2.64}$ (f) $25\overline{)1.75}$

(g) $75\overline{)1.575}$ (h) $25\overline{)75.25}$ (i) $47\overline{)317.72}$ (j) $64\overline{)131.2}$

To divide a decimal by a decimal, move the decimal point of the divisor to the right until the divisor becomes a whole number; then move the decimal point in the dividend the same number of places, adding zeros if necessary; then place the decimal point in the quotient. Finally, divide as one would with whole numbers.

Example: 4.5 ÷ .15

$$\begin{array}{r} 30. \\ .15.\overline{)4.50.} \end{array}$$

The decimal point in the divisor and the dividend is moved two places to the right.

Practice Set V - 11

Divide:

1) Divide 9801.9 by 0.9

2) Divide 892.5 by 7.0

3) Divide 58.32 by 1.8

4) Divide 17.28 by 0.12

5) Divide 5.12 by 0.08

6) Divide 3.43 by 0.7

7) Divide 306.72 by 0.8

8) Divide 793.1 by 0.07

9) Divide 100.1 by 0.001

10) Divide 795.07 by 4.3

11) $.0075\overline{).6}$

12) $.25\overline{)75.25}$

13) $4.7\overline{)317.72}$

14) $6.4\overline{)873.42}$

You have divided decimals into whole numbers, whole numbers into decimals, and decimals into decimals. Next, lots of practice in placing the decimal point.

Practice Set V - 12

Location of decimal point

The answer for each of the following contains the digits 343. You must correctly place the decimal point in the answer, adding zeros where necessary. The first couple are done for you as examples. It is not necessary to actually do the division.

(1) $124\overline{)42.532}$ — answer: .343

(2) $124\overline{)425.32}$ — answer: 3.43

(3) $1.24\overline{)42.532}$

(4) $.124\overline{)425.32}$

(5) $12.4\overline{)4253.2}$

(6) $12.4\overline{).42532}$

(7) $1.24\overline{)4253.2}$

(8) $124\overline{).42532}$

(9) $.124\overline{).42532}$

(10) $12.4\overline{)4.2532}$

(11) $1.24\overline{).042532}$

(12) $12.4\overline{)42.532}$

(13) $0.124\overline{)4253.2}$

(14) $0.124\overline{).042532}$

(15) $.00124\overline{).0042532}$

(19) $124\overline{)42532}$

(20) $.124\overline{)42.532}$

(21) $.124\overline{)4.2532}$

(22) $.0124\overline{).042532}$

(23) $.124\overline{).42532}$

(24) $.124\overline{).00042532}$

(25) $12{,}400\overline{).42532}$

(26) $12{,}400\overline{)42{,}532}$

(27) $124\overline{).0042532}$

(28) $1240\overline{).0042532}$

(29) $1240\overline{)4.2532}$

(30) $12400\overline{)42532}$

(31) $.124\overline{)42.532}$

(32) $1.24\overline{)42.532}$

(33) $12.4\overline{).0042532}$

Practice Set V - 13 Review

I. Perform the indicated operation:

(a) $\begin{array}{r} 0.315 \\ \times 3.12 \\ \hline \end{array}$

(b) $\begin{array}{r} 9.10 \\ \times 9.1 \\ \hline \end{array}$

(c) $\begin{array}{r} 56.7 \\ \times 0.42 \\ \hline \end{array}$

(d) $\begin{array}{r} 0.096 \\ \times 7.8 \\ \hline \end{array}$

(e) $\begin{array}{r} 357.1 \\ \times 0.111 \\ \hline \end{array}$

(f) $\begin{array}{r} 5.03 \\ \times 0.9111 \\ \hline \end{array}$

(g) $\begin{array}{r} 2.56 \\ \times 0.48 \\ \hline \end{array}$

(h) $\begin{array}{r} 600.73 \\ \times 1.12 \\ \hline \end{array}$

(i) $\begin{array}{r} 1.512 \\ \times 1.34 \\ \hline \end{array}$

(j) $\begin{array}{r} 2.432 \\ \times .07 \\ \hline \end{array}$

(k) $\begin{array}{r} 0.431 \\ \times 0.32 \\ \hline \end{array}$

(l) $\begin{array}{r} 7.62 \\ \times 3.1 \\ \hline \end{array}$

(m) 8.031 ×1.34	(n) 1.213 ×0.561	(o) 2.521 ×6.21	(p) 7.36 ×.62
(q) 2.5 ×2.1	(r) 9.16 ×1.72	(s) 15.4 ×1.2	(t) 0.0786 ×2.4
(u) 14.807 ×4.1	(v) 89.7 ×5.3	(w) 15.4 ×70	(x) 98.23 ×100
(y) 14.887 ×0.1	(z) 22.73 ×0.01	(aa) 17.1 ×0.001	(bb) 12.89 ×0.0001

II. Solve:

(a) 1.8 ÷ 0.002

(b) 1.616 ÷ 0.77

(c) 76.4 ÷ 38.2

(d) 98.65 ÷ 13.1

(e) 3.6503 ÷ 1.25

(f) 9.9 ÷ 3.3

(g) 0.567 ÷ 14

(h) 3.693 ÷ 0.03

(i) 50.25 ÷ 0.5

(j) 200 ÷ 2.5

(k) 5.40 ÷ 0.6

(l) 24.57 ÷ 2.7

(m) 7.5 ÷ 1.5

(n) 0.006 ÷ 0.003

(o) 84.84 ÷ 4.2

(s) $98.3525 \div 1000$

(t) $8.359 \div 0.1$

(u) $8.359 \div 0.01$

(v) $8.359 \div 0.001$

(w) $5.40 \div 0.01$

(x) $24.56 \div 0.03$

Often, while doing lab work, a need arises to divide by ten, or one hundred, 1000, one tenth, one hundredth, or so on. Like multiplying by powers of ten, dividing by powers of ten also can be short cut.

Example: Divide 2.4 by each of the following . . .

$2.4 \div 10 = .24$

$2.4 \div 0.1 = 24$

$2.4 \div 100 = .024$

$2.4 \div 0.01 = 240$

$2.4 \div 1000 = .0024$

$2.4 \div 0.001 = 2400$

In the example above, when we divided 2.4 by 10, how did the decimal point change?

____

You should have noticed that the decimal point moved one place to the left in the quotient when dividing by ten. When we divided by 0.001 the decimal point moved three places to the right in the quotient. Can you think of a rule that governs this behavior?

Practice Set V - 14

Divide.

1) $0.01\overline{)314.2}$

2) $1000\overline{)314.2}$

3) $10\overline{)314.2}$

4) $0.001\overline{)3.142}$

5) $100\overline{)31.42}$

6) $0.0001\overline{)314.2}$

7) 314.2 divided by 10,000

8) 0.3142 divided by 0.1

9) 100,000 divided into 314.2

10) 0.000001 divided into 3.142

The following practice set involves multiplying and dividing by powers of ten. This relationship will be further explored with scientific notation later in this chapter. Try using some short cut method when possible.

Practice Set V - 15 Perform the indicated operation relocating the decimal point as indicated.

Multiply	*Divide*
(a) $231 \times 10 =$	$231 \div 10 =$
(b) 2001×0.0001	$2001 \div 0.0001$
(c) 48.236×1000	$48.236 \div 1000$
(d) 2.310×0.01	$2.310 \div 0.01$
(e) 4.691×100	$4.691 \div 100$
(f) 96.39×1000	$96.39 \div 1000$

(g) 856.9×0.0001 $856.9 \div 0.0001$

(h) 9.8751×0.001 $9.8751 \div 0.001$

(i) 18.754×10 $18.754 \div 10$

(j) 910.4×100 $910.4 \div 100$

(k) 876.12×1000 $876.12 \div 1000$

(l) 9543.1×0.001 $9543.1 \div 0.001$

(m) 0.998×0.1 $0.998 \div 0.1$

(n) 576.24×0.0001 $576.24 \div 0.0001$

(o) 5.1×0.01 $5.1 \div 0.01$

(p) 79.99×1 $79.99 \div 1$

(q) 85.333×10000 $85.333 \div 10000$

(r) 94.999×0.01 $94.999 \div 0.01$

(s) 87.666×0.001 $87.666 \div 0.001$

(t) 87.632×0.001 $87.632 \div 0.001$

(u) 994.33×0.00001 $994.33 \div 0.00001$

(v) 8643.2×10 $8643.2 \div 10$

(w) 99.999×10000 $99.999 \div 10000$

(x) 87.432×0.001 $87.432 \div 0.001$

(y) 8.7432×0.01 $87.432 \div 0.01$

(z) 954.11×0.0001 $954.11 \div 0.0001$

(aa) 87.654×100 $87.654 \div 100$

Scientific Notation

To convert scientific notation from a decimal

- based on powers of ten
- Format: $N \times 10^x$ where $1 \leq N < 10$ and x is any integer

Easy to convert by simply moving the decimal point:

- for a number greater than one (1)

← move the decimal point the required "steps" to the Left The number of steps represents x and x is positive.

- for a number less than 1

→ move the decimal point the required steps to the Right. The number of steps represents x and x is negative.

Here's how it works …

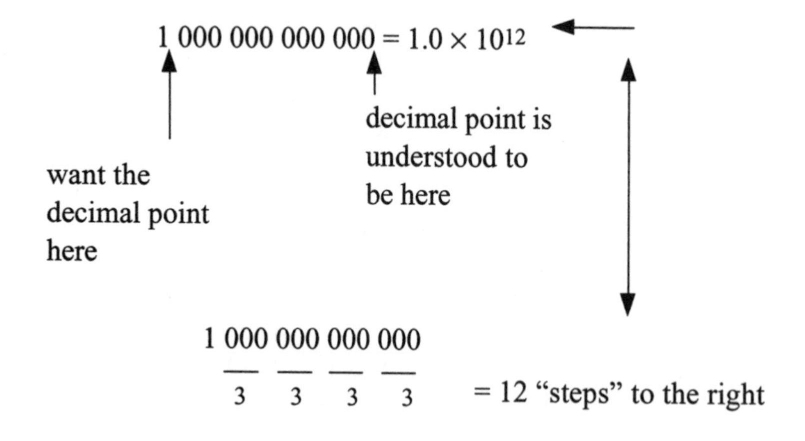

… this gives the desired **N** such that **N** is (at least) 1.0 and the power of ten corresponds to the number of places ("steps") taken!

Examples:

$1000 = 1.0 \times 10^3$ $1520 = 1.52 \times 10^3$ $0.003 = 3 \times 10^{-3}$

$0.00415 = 4.15 \times 10^{-3}$ $10004000 = 1.0004 \times 10^7$

$0.0000045 = 4.5 \times 10^{-6}$ $1\ 000\ 000\ 000\ 000 = 1.0 \times 10^{12}$

To a decimal from scientific notation

The sign (positive/negative) of the exponent of ten (10^X) determines the direction to move when converting from scientific notation to standard numbers.

- if the sign of the exponent is negative move the decimal that many places Left
- if the sign of the exponent is positive, move the decimal point to the Right

Examples:

$1.4 \times 10^3 = 1400$ $2.0 \times 10^5 = 200000$ $3.1 \times 10^{-4} = 0.00031$

$9.5 \times 10^{-7} = 0.00000095$ $4.3 \times 10^2 = 430$

$4.5 \times 10^{-6} = 0.0000045$

move decimal point 6 places to the left (since minus)

Rounding Decimals

Sometimes, it is necessary to express an answer correct to the nearest hundredth or to the nearest thousandth, for example. After finding the solution, the answer may be rewritten with as many decimal places as are required to bring it to the degree of accuracy determined by the problem. This process is known as rounding off a number. Rounding off means expressing a decimal with fewer digits. The answer should be carried out one more place than the accuracy calls for, then "rounded" as indicated by that digit. Round to the nearest hundredth means the answer should have two decimal places. Thus, the answer should be carried to three places and the answer rounded off to two places. If the digit to the right of the place we are rounding is 5 or more, drop it and add one to the digit in the preceding place. If the digit is less than 5, drop it and do not change the preceding digit.

Example: Round .671 to the nearest hundredth. Since the third decimal place (thousandths) is a 1, drop that and do not change the preceding digit (the 7) - the answer is then .67.

Round .876 to the nearest hundredth.

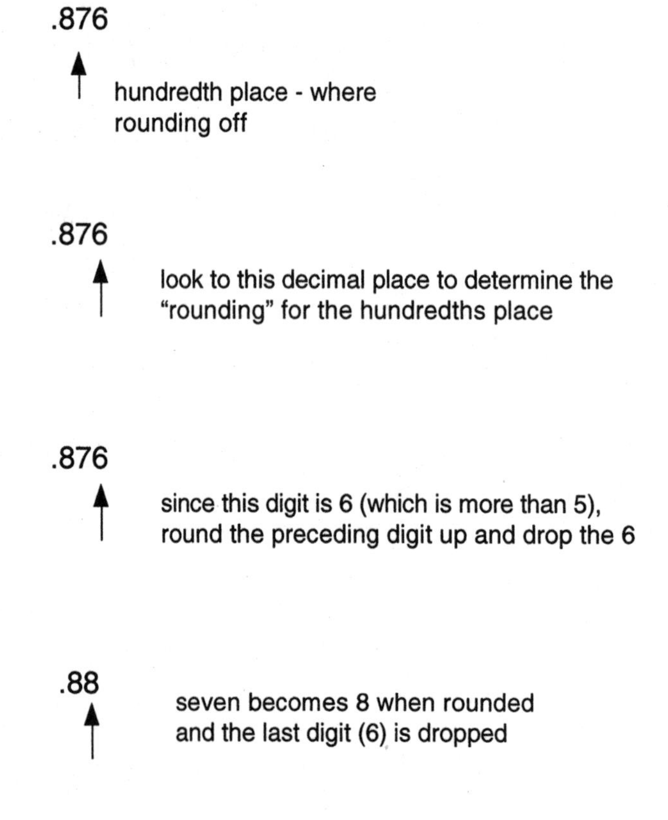

.876 rounded to the nearest hundredth is .88

You try it! Round .7536 to the nearest thousandth. (answer: 0.754)

Practice Set V - 16

Round each of the following to the nearest .001

(a) .8731 (b) .7899 (c) .7777

(d) .6312 (e) .6214 (f) .7325

Round each of the following to the nearest .01

(a) .654 (b) .667 (c) .372

(d) .982 (e) .427 (f) .635

Practice Set V - 17

Solve each of the following. Find the quotient to the nearest hundredth. (This means you'll need to carry your answer to three decimal places in order to round.)

(a) $29.7 \div 4 =$ (b) $3.8 \div 51$

(c) $48.1 \div 23$ (d) $0.0734 \div 5$

(e) $100 \div 21$

(f) $572.6 \div 921$

(g) $56.43 \div 3.1$

(h) $100 \div 3183$

(i) $234 \div 0.065$

(j) $345.9 \div 0.21$

(k) $1 \div 3$

(l) $1 \div 6$

Solve the following. Express the answer to the nearest thousandth.

(a) $457.1 \div 0.83$

(b) $63.75 \div 4.6$

(c) $82.3 \div 3.1416$

(d) $4 \div 0.3183$

(e) $80.70 \div 27.7$

(f) $807 \div 255$

(g) $236.6 \div 7.3$

(h) $500.9 \div 20.3$

(i) $45.843 \div 21$

(j) $66 \div 25$

(k) $0.48 \div 0.13$

(l) $1 \div 7$

Practice Set V - 18

I. Round to the indicated (by underline) place.

(a) $5\underline{8}9$ (b) $0.003\underline{2}9$ (c) $17\underline{5}9$

(d) $0.\underline{8}428$ (e) $1\underline{6}07$ (f) $0.8\underline{5}49$

(g) $19\underline{0}5$ (h) $0.\underline{0}02$ (i) $10\underline{6}6$

(j) $1.9\underline{8}08$ (k) $\underline{5}1$ (l) $4.\underline{5}49$

(m) $14\underline{3}2$ (n) $1.4\underline{3}2$ (o) $876\underline{9}29$

(p) $8.\underline{5}76$ (q) $48\underline{9}9902$ (r) $0.0\underline{3}47$

II. Express each of the following in scientific notation.

(a) 100,000 (b) 100 (c) 1,000,000 (d) 0.0001

(e) 0.00000001 (f) 0.01 (g) 0.0000000001 (h) 0.000001

(i) 1000 (j) 10,000,000

III. Rewrite each of the following from scientific notation to whole number or decimal notation.

(a) 10^6 (b) 10^4 (c) 10^3 (d) 10^7

(e) 10^{-3} (f) 10^{-5} (g) 10^{-2}

(h) 10^{-6} (i) 10^2

Practice Set V - 19

Convert to/from scientific notation.

(a) 2×10^4 (b) 8.4×10^6

(c) 0.33×10^{-2} (d) 0.33×10^2

(e) 8.47×10^{-8} (f) 0.00035

(g) 0.000839

(h) 10857

(i) 87.69×10^{8}

(j) 4.235×10^{-4}

(k) 6.798×10^{-7}

(l) 246810

(m) 0.00357

(n) 8.276×10^{-5}

(o) 7.5×10^{-6}

(p) 15×10^{-6}

(q) 4×10^{7}

(r) 0.0000436

(s) 45789

(t) 257

(u) 8324.67

(v) 2.69×10^{4}

(w) 0.00357

(x) 0.00005

(y) 4.83

(z) 0.00001

Fraction Review

1. Add and reduce to lowest terms:

(a) $2\frac{3}{9}$, $1\frac{1}{27}$, $\frac{6}{18}$, $+\ \frac{1}{3}$

(b) $5\frac{1}{8}$, $2\frac{3}{64}$, $\frac{3}{24}$, $+\ 3\frac{4}{16}$

(c) $6\frac{1}{4}$, $\frac{5}{6}$, $12\frac{5}{8}$, $+\ \frac{12}{32}$

(d) $5\frac{6}{8}$, $6\frac{1}{4}$, $12\frac{1}{6}$, $+\ 1\frac{3}{8}$

(e) $\frac{7}{8}$, $\frac{3}{4}$, $+\ \frac{9}{10}$

2. Which fraction is largest? Circle the correct choice.

(a) $\frac{5}{8}$ or $\frac{3}{4}$

(b) $\frac{15}{20}$ or $\frac{10}{12}$

(c) $\frac{5}{6}$ or $\frac{2}{3}$

(d) $\frac{1}{8}$ or $\frac{1}{6}$

(e) $\frac{1}{16}$ or $\frac{3}{4}$

(f) $\frac{7}{9}$ or $\frac{9}{10}$

(g) $\frac{1}{2}$ or $\frac{2}{3}$

(h) $\frac{5}{11}$ or $\frac{1}{3}$

3. Convert to mixed or whole numbers. Reduce and express in lowest terms.

(a) $\frac{20}{5} =$ (b) $\frac{16}{5} =$ (c) $\frac{50}{6} =$ (d) $\frac{13}{12} =$ (e) $\frac{36}{12} =$

(f) $\frac{56}{6} =$ (g) $\frac{42}{3} =$ (h) $\frac{19}{4} =$ (i) $\frac{72}{8} =$ (j) $\frac{7}{2} =$

4. Multiply. Reduce to lowest terms:

(a) $\frac{2}{3} \times \frac{5}{12} =$

(b) $1\frac{1}{4} \times 5\frac{1}{8} =$

(c) $2\frac{1}{2} \times 3\frac{2}{3} \times 4\frac{5}{8} =$

(d) $\frac{7}{9} \times \frac{1}{5} =$

(e) $2\frac{3}{5} \times 4\frac{1}{5} =$

(f) $\frac{24}{25} \times \frac{11}{20} =$

(g) $1\frac{3}{4} \times 2\frac{3}{4} =$

(h) $3\frac{3}{4} \times 1\frac{3}{5} \times 2\frac{4}{5} =$

(i) $\frac{1}{3} \times 4\frac{1}{2} =$

(j) $\frac{5}{12} \times \frac{2}{3} =$

(k) $3\frac{1}{6} \times 3\frac{1}{4} =$

(l) $\frac{3}{4} \times \frac{2}{5} =$

(m) $6\frac{1}{2} \times 4\frac{7}{8} =$

(n) $\frac{3}{5} \times \frac{3}{2} =$

(o) $8\frac{2}{5} \times 2\frac{3}{5} =$

(p) $\frac{5}{8} \times \frac{4}{5} =$

(q) $2\frac{1}{3} \times 4\frac{5}{12} =$

(r) $12\frac{1}{2} \times 17\frac{1}{3} \times 3\frac{3}{4} =$

5. Subtract and reduce to lowest terms:

(a) $\frac{7}{8} - \frac{1}{4}$

(b) $5\frac{4}{5} - 2\frac{3}{5}$

(c) $12\frac{1}{2} - 2\frac{1}{6}$

(d) $\frac{9}{10} - \frac{3}{5}$

(e) $15\frac{2}{3} - 3\frac{2}{3}$

(f) $\dfrac{7}{10} - \dfrac{2}{5}$

(g) $\dfrac{11}{16} - \dfrac{1}{2}$

(h) $19\dfrac{1}{2} - 11\dfrac{1}{4}$

(i) $61\dfrac{2}{3} - 2\dfrac{4}{5}$

(j) $1\dfrac{1}{2} - \dfrac{3}{4}$

6. Divide. Reduce to lowest terms:

(a) $8\dfrac{5}{8} \div \dfrac{1}{50} =$

(b) $\dfrac{4}{75} \div \dfrac{7}{25} =$

(c) $12\dfrac{4}{5} \div 5\dfrac{1}{2} =$

(d) $25\dfrac{1}{2} \div 7\dfrac{3}{4} =$

(e) $\dfrac{3}{20} \div \dfrac{1}{2} =$

(f) $\dfrac{4}{25} \div \dfrac{8}{25} =$

(g) $190\dfrac{3}{4} \div 2\dfrac{5}{8} =$

(h) $4\dfrac{1}{5} \div 2\dfrac{9}{10} =$

(i) $1\dfrac{1}{2} \div \dfrac{3}{4} =$

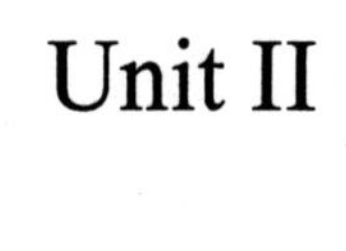
Unit II

Chapter 6

Miscellaneous

Objectives

Upon completion, the student must be able to do the following:

- **Recognize Greek letters used in Medicine and the Sciences.**
- **Be familiar with definitions of geometry used in the lab.**
- **Know the parts of a syringe and different types of syringes.**
- **Understand terms frequently encountered in a laboratory.**

The Greek Alphabet

Α	α	alpha
Β	β	beta
Γ	γ	gamma
Δ	δ	delta
Ε	ε	epsilon
Ζ	ζ	zeta
Η	η	eta
Θ	θ	theta
Ι	ι	iota
Κ	κ	kappa
Λ	λ	lambda
Μ	μ	mu
Ν	ν	nu
Ξ	ξ	xi
Ο	ο	omicron
Π	π	pi
Ρ	ρ	rho
Σ	σ	sigma
Τ	τ	tau
Υ	υ	upsilon
Φ	φ	phi
Χ	χ	chi
Ψ	ψ	psi
Ω	ω	omega

After learning the symbols, complete the chart that follows.

Practice Set VI - 1

(a)	______	______	alpha
(b)	B	______	________
(c)	______	_______	pi
(d)	________	________	gamma
(e)	________	________	sigma
(f)	M	__________	__________
(g)	Θ	__________	____________
(h)	Ω	_________	____________
(i)	__________	δ	_____________
(j)	___________	__________	lambda

Geometry Terms

a. *Parallel:* two or more lines in the same plane, which extend in the same direction, are everywhere equidistant and never meet. The symbol for parallel is ||. *Example:* when administering an intramuscular (IM) injection in the leg, the angle of the needle is parallel to the femur.

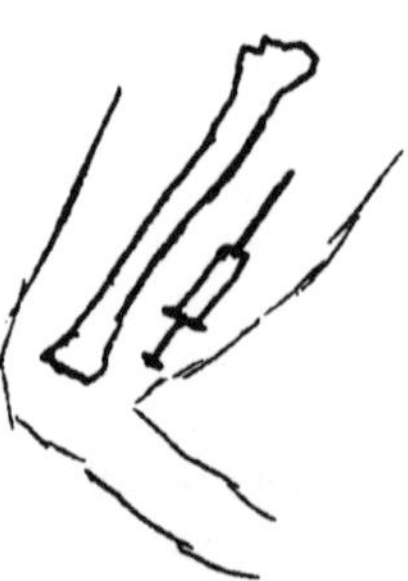

b. *Perpendicular:* two lines which intersect at exactly 90° . The angle formed is often referred to as a right angle. The symbol is ⊥

c. *Concentric circles* are different sized circles having a common center.

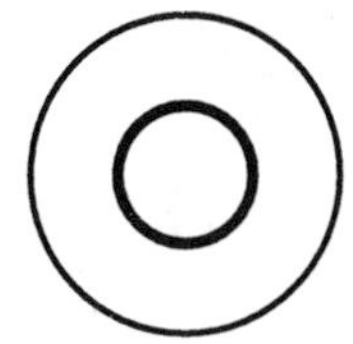

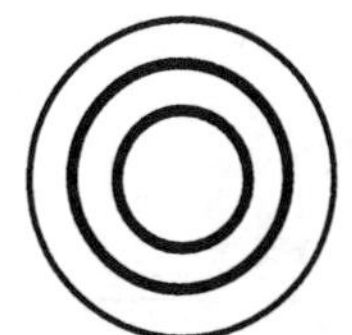

Syringes often have tips places in a concentric manner.

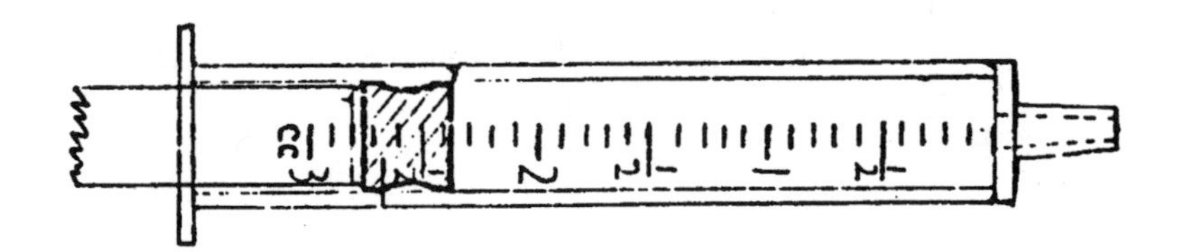

d. *Eccentric circles* are two circles in the same plane which do not have the same center.

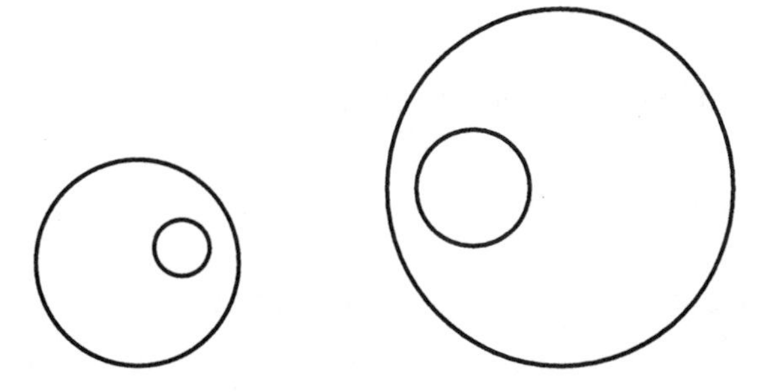

Syringes are also found with eccentrically placed tips.

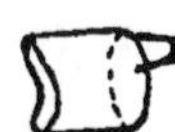

The parts of a syringe:

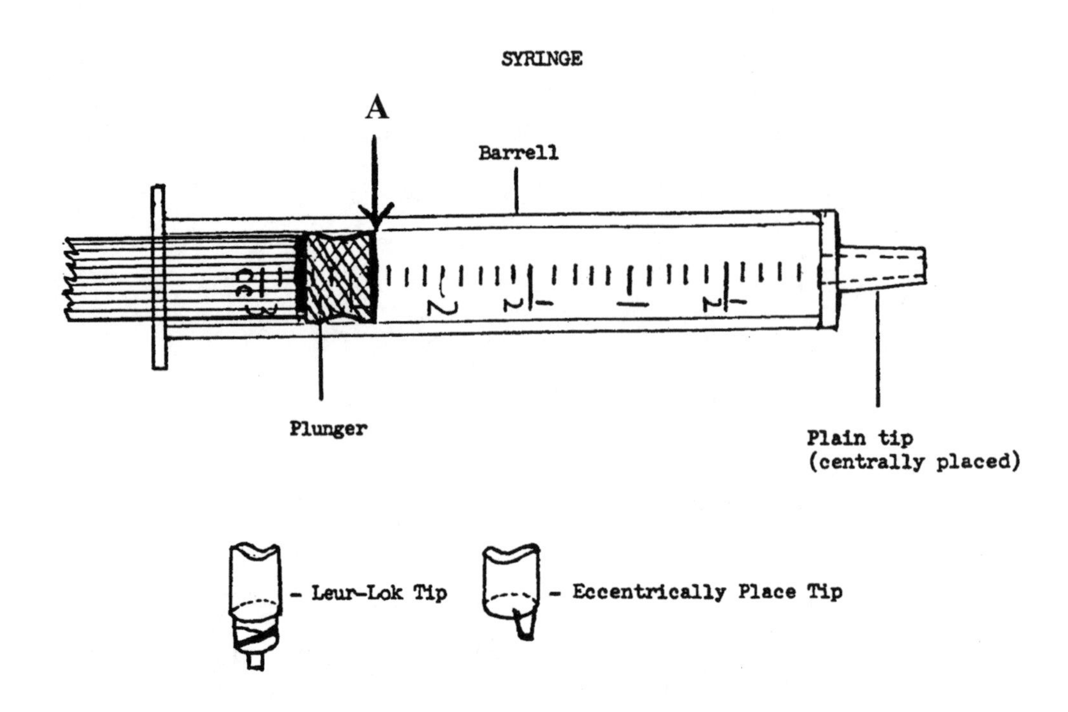

1. Syringes are usually measured in cc (cubic centimeters).

2. A cc is the same measure as a ml (milliliter).

3. Syringes are occasionally marked in types of units besides cc.

4. The plunger moves up and down inside the barrel. The quantity within the syringe is read from the scale where the leading edge of the plunger touches the barrel. (See A in picture of parts of a syringe.)

e. Degrees of a circle: Each circle is divided into 360 degrees.

The number of degrees in a quarter circle is 90°. Ninety degrees makes a right angle.

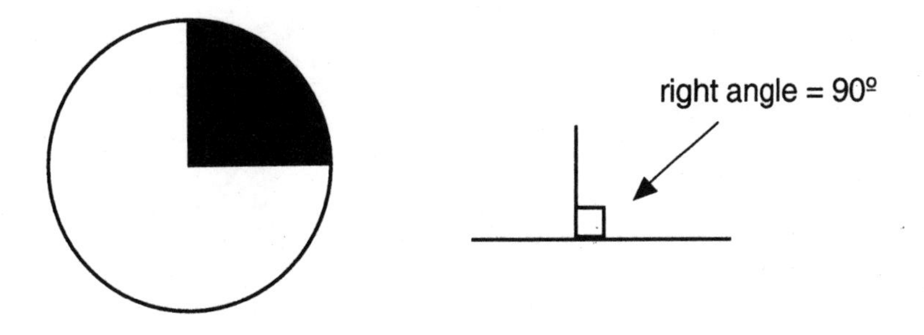

Practice Set VI - 2

(a) Identify:

The lines shown are _____________________.

(b) α α is called a _________________ angle and the two lines are

_________________________ to one another

(c) Name the type of each circle set shown:

(i) ______________________ (ii) __________________________

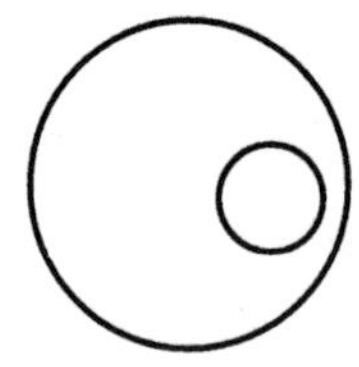

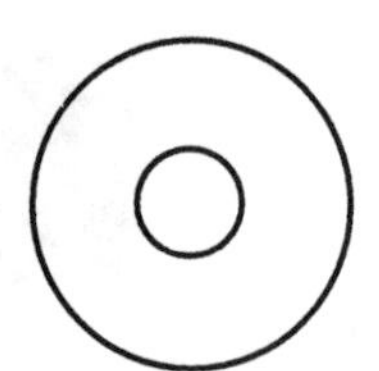

(d) Name the parts of the syringe:

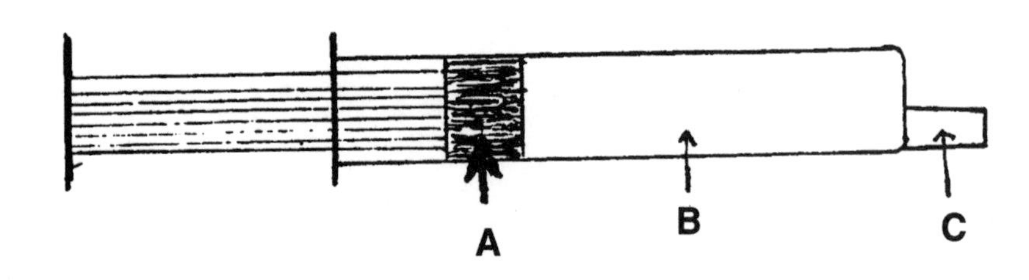

A. _______________ B. _______________ C. _______________

Indicate the placement of the item at letter C: ________________________________

(e) A circle is divided into ________________ degrees.

(f) Estimate the number of degrees indicated by each drawing:

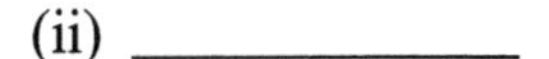

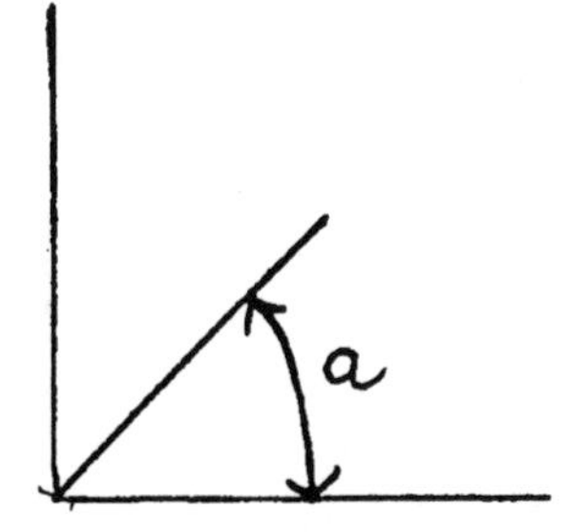

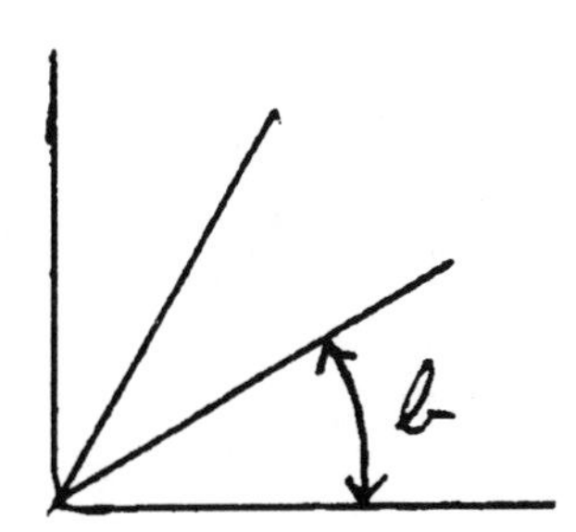

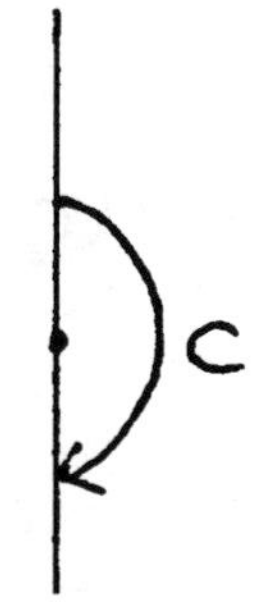

Additional terms with which the technician should be familiar include the following.

Parallax is the apparent displacement of an object when viewed from two different points.

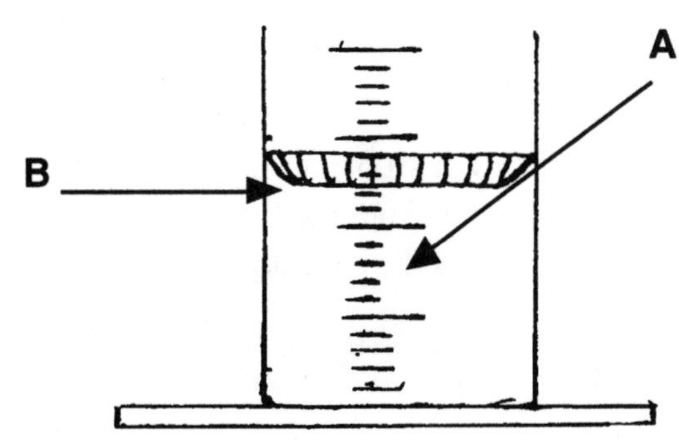

View from A and B is different. The view from A causes an incorrect reading!

Meniscus - a liquid wets the container it is in and causes a rise along the contact surface. The portion of the liquid not in contact with the surface does not rise. The result is a curved upper surface of a liquid column (as shown.)

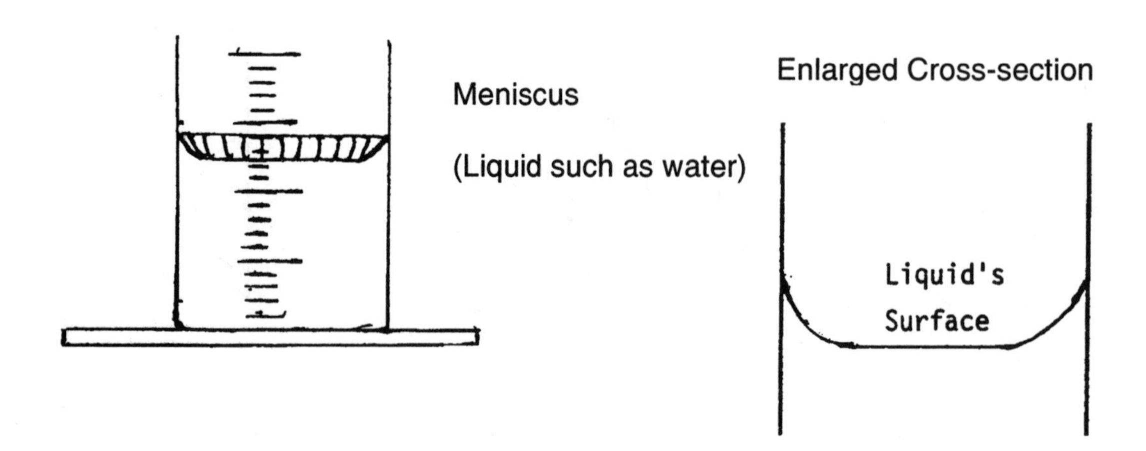

Reading a graduated cylinder with meniscus can result in an error in measurement. Always read straight across the cylinder, lining up the marked measurements along the outside of the cylinder with the bottom of the meniscus.

A similar error can occur when reading instrument scales. If a scale is viewed off-center, the reading may be distorted.

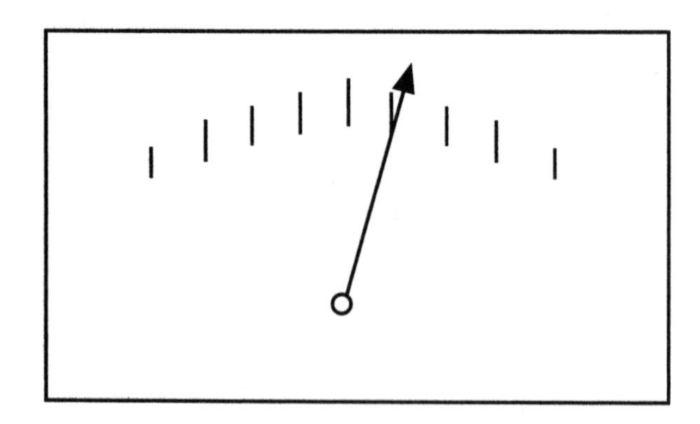

Read instrument scales carefully. Read directly from the front and at the same level as the instrument.

Capillary action is the effect of a liquid being pulled up in a fine bore tube higher than its level in the surrounding liquid. The finer the bore of the tube, the higher the liquid will be pulled.

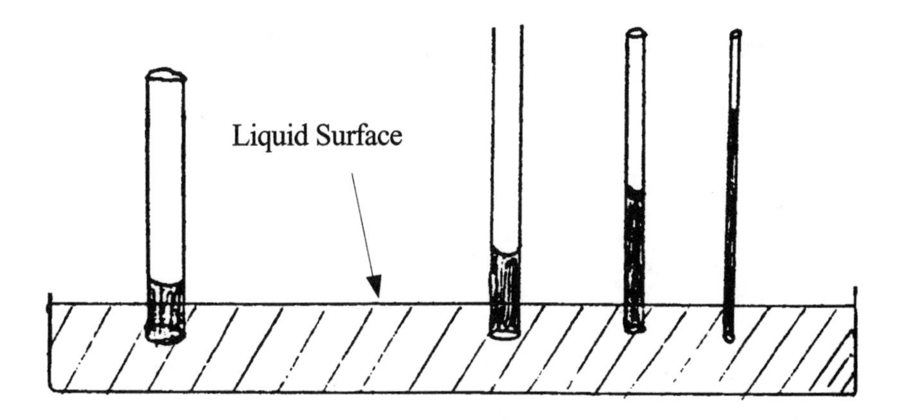

Density is defined as the amount of mass (or weight) per unit volume. For example,

$$\frac{grams}{milliliter} \qquad \frac{kilogram}{liter} \qquad \frac{lbs}{foot^3}$$

abbreviations can include: g/ml, g/cc, kg/L, lb/ft^3

The density of lead is greater than water; following are some common densities for water, wood, gasoline, and urine.

Densities

	g/cc	lb/cubic foot
water	1.000	62.400
wood	0.900	58.500
gasoline	0.860	53.800
urine	1.035	- - -

Specific gravity is a means of comparing densities to that of water. Note that specific gravity is a number with no units.

$$\text{Specific gravity} = \frac{\text{Density of a substance}}{\text{Density of water}}$$

Examples:

(1)

$$\text{Specific gravity of Lead} = \frac{11.3 \text{ g / cc}}{1 \text{ g / cc}} = 11.3$$

(2)

$$\text{Specific gravity of urine} = \frac{1.035 \text{ g / cc}}{1 \text{ g / cc}} = 1.035$$

Practice Set VI - 3

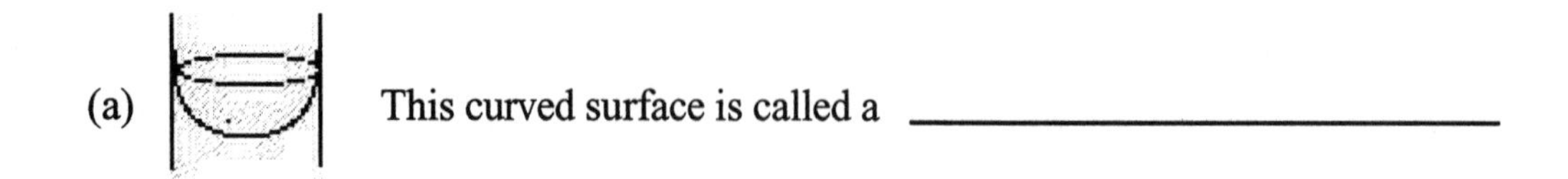

(a) This curved surface is called a ______________________

(b) Water can be pulled up a fine bore tube by ______________________

(c) 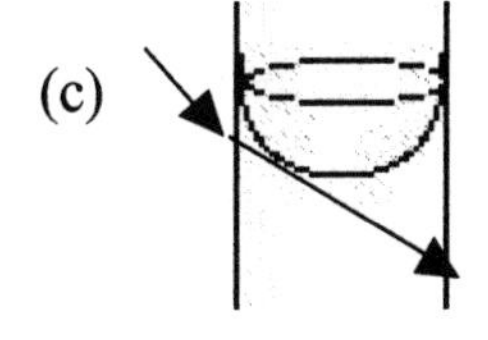

Misreading of the liquid level (as shown) is caused by

____

(d) Define Density:

(e) The density of water is: ______________ g / cc or ______________ lb / ft^3 .

(f) Define specific gravity:

Brief Introduction to the Metric System

The metric system will be covered in detail in Chapter 10; however, for now, it's a good idea to begin to familiarize yourself with the basics of the metric system.

The metric system is based upon multiples of ten. Its base units are the meter for length, the gram for weight, and the liter for volume. The system uses prefixes to differentiate among smaller and larger units. The chart following shows the basics of the system. You should learn to recreate this chart on demand. Learn the terms and equivalents of the various prefixes. Note the factors, or powers, of ten that distinguish units. For example, a kilogram is 1000 grams. A milliliter is one-thousandth of a liter; there are 1000 milliliters in a liter!

One more example: 5000 milliliters equals ?? kiloliters? From milliliters to kiloliters is six steps to the left. Move the decimal at the end of 5000 milliliters to the left six places to get .005 kiloliters!

To change units, one need only move the decimal point to the right or left depending on whether the units that are being changed are larger or smaller than the desired units. With this chart, you need only count the "steps" from the initial units to the desired units. Move the decimal the same number of places as "steps" in the same direction you moved on the chart. For example, to change from hectometers to centimeters requires moving four steps to the right. So, to change 5.2 hectometers to centimeters move the decimal point four places to the right to achieve 52, 000. centimeters. Thus, 5.2 hectometers equals 52, 000 centimeters!

For a full-size version of the chart being discussed see page 105

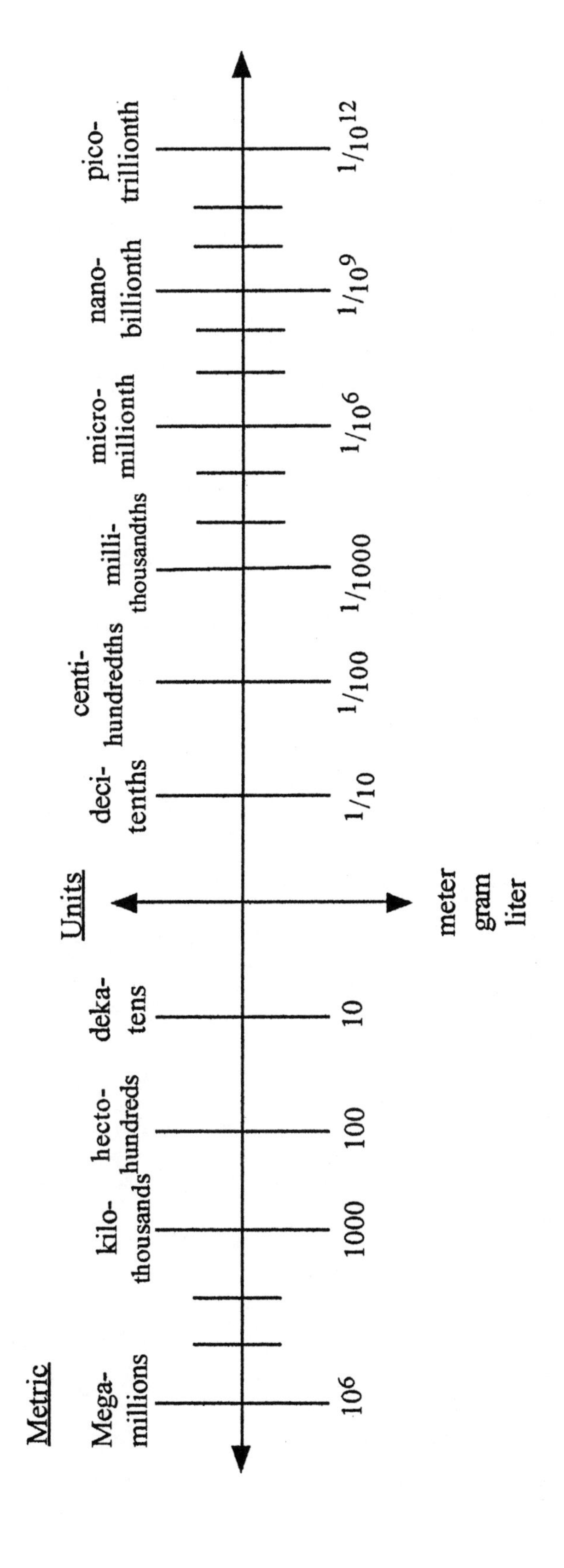
Metric
Mega-
millions
10^6
kilo-
thousands
1000
hecto-
hundreds
100
deka-
tens
10
Units
meter
gram
liter
deci-
tenths
$1/10$
centi-
hundredths
$1/100$
milli-
thousandths
$1/1000$
micro-
millionth
$1/10^6$
nano-
billionth
$1/10^9$
pico-
trillionth
$1/10^{12}$

Chapter 7

Percentage

Objectives

Upon completion, the student must be able to do the following:

- **Change a decimal to a percent.**
- **Change a percent to a decimal.**
- **Change a fraction to a percent.**
- **Change a percent to a common fraction.**
- **Determine the percentage of a given number.**
- **Determine what percent one number is of another.**
- **Change values to and from gram per deciliter.**

There is a need to know how to compute percentage in business and industry. Many handbooks, manuals, and catalogs make references to percents. The sign, or symbol, for percent is %. Percent means *per hundred.* Per means divide, and cent refers to 100; thus, percent means something divided by 100. 40% is read forty percent and indicates 40 hundredths or 40 parts out of 100.

Changing Percent to a Number

Math operations involving percentages cannot use the symbol %. We must first change the percent into a decimal or common fraction. Since percent means hundredths, we can change percent into a decimal. Recall that hundredths is two (decimal) places to the right of the decimal point. In a whole number, the decimal is understood to be at the rightmost place of the number.

Examples: 8 is the same as 8.0

97 is the same as 97.0

When multiplying a number by 100, we learned to move the decimal point two places to the right. [Recall scientific notation where $10^2 = 100$]. If dividing by 100, move the decimal two places to the left. Percent means divide by 100; therefore, to change a percent to a decimal, drop the % sign and move the decimal two places to the left.

Examples: a. 81% = .81

b. 96% = .96

c. 5% = .05

d. 112% = 1.12

Practice Set VII - 1

Change the following % to decimals:

1) 15%

2) 33%

3) 40%

4) 1%

5) 9%

6) 125%

7) 94.3%

8) 100%

9) 5%

To change a decimal to a percent, do the opposite. To change a decimal to a percent requires us to move the decimal point two places to the right and append the percent sign, %.

Examples: .12 = 12%

.07 = 7%

1.19 = 119%

Practice Set VII - 2

Change the following decimals to percent:

1) .10 =
5) 6.3 =
9) .9 =

2) .12 =
6) .762 =
10) .375 =

3) .125 =
7) .875 =
11) .085 =

4) .09 =
8) 2.25 =
12) .1 =

To change from a percent to a common fraction requires expressing the value of the percent as a fraction rather than a decimal. To do this, use the value of the percent as the numerator and 100 as the denominator. Reduce as necessary.

Examples: $21\% = \frac{21}{100}$ $40\% = \frac{40}{100} = \frac{2}{5}$ $75\% = \frac{75}{100} = \frac{3}{4}$

Practice Set VII - 3

Change the given percents to common fractions: (Be sure to reduce)

1) 60% =
3) 10% =
5) 110% =

2) 50% =
4) 8% =
6) 90% =

To change any fraction to percent, first change the fraction to a decimal by dividing the denominator into the numerator. Then change the resulting decimal to a percent as previously discussed. (See Practice Set VII - 2.)

Examples: Change $\frac{1}{2}$ to percent $2\overline{)1.0}$ with quotient $.5$: $= 0.5 = 50\%$

and $^{3}/_{8}$ as a percent:

$$\frac{3}{8} = 8\overline{)3.000} = 37.5\% \quad (\text{quotient } .375)$$

Practice Set VII - 4

Change the following fractions to percents:

1) $\frac{1}{4} =$

2) $\frac{3}{5} =$

3) $\frac{7}{10} =$

4) $\frac{1}{12} =$

5) $\frac{3}{16} =$

6) $\frac{7}{8} =$

7) $\frac{5}{6} =$

8) $\frac{1}{5} =$

Practice Set VII - 5

I. Express each of the following percents as a decimal:

1) 2.5%

2) 8.5%

3) 7.11%

4) 6.25%

5) 9.5%

6) 190%

II. Express each of the following decimals as a percent:

7) 0.33

8) 0.3633

9) 0.987

10) 0.63

11) 0.11

12) 16.375

III. Express each of the following fractions to the nearest tenth of a percent:

13) $\frac{1}{8}$

14) $\frac{5}{8}$

15) $\frac{1}{7}$

16) $\frac{4}{7}$

17) $\frac{1}{9}$

18) $\frac{5}{9}$

19) $\frac{1}{11}$

20) $\frac{7}{11}$

IV. Express each of the following percents as a common fraction and reduce to lowest terms where necessary:

21) 2%

22) 8%

23) 20%

24) 40%

25) 32%

26) 48%

27) 38.5%

28) 1.75%

V. Express each of the following as (a) a percent, (b) as a decimal and (c) a fraction or mixed number:

29) 8%

30) 7.5%

31) 0.925

32) 66.7%

33) $\frac{3}{7}$

34) 0.125

35) 650.00

36) $\frac{9}{16}$

37) 125%

38) $\frac{11}{42}$

39) 0.333

40) $3\frac{5}{8}$

41) $1\frac{5}{9}$

42) 3.25%

Now that we know the mechanics of changing percents to decimals and fractions and back again, we can use that knowledge to solve problems involving percentages. To find the percent of a given number use the following guidelines:

Guide for finding any percent of a number

- Convert the percent to either a fractional or decimal equivalent.
- Multiply the given number by this equivalent.
- Label answer with appropriate unit of measure.

Example 1: Find 16% of 1218 millimeters.

Step 1: Change 16% to a decimal   16% = .16

Step 2: Multiply

$$\begin{array}{r} 1218 \\ \underline{\times .16} \\ 194.88 \end{array}$$

Step 3: Label answer: 194.88 millimeters

Example 2: Follow the same steps when the percent is a mixed number.

Find $6\ ^1/_4$ % of 782 hours

Step 1: $6\ ^1/_4\ \% = 6.25\% = 0.0625$

Step 2:

$$\begin{array}{r} 782 \\ \underline{\times .0625} \\ 48.8750 \end{array}$$

Step 3: 48.875 hours

Here's another way to think about percentage problems…

consider the sentence…

What percent of something is this?

(1) × (2) = (3)

There are three "parts" here. Also, **of** means "times" and **is** means "equals". You will always know (or be able to determine) two of the parts. Part 1 is the percentage; Parts 2 and 3 are the numbers. Thus, there are three possibilities:

What percent of something is this?

	①	×	②	=	③	
(1) 35% of 52 is ? In this case, the model is	35%	×	52	=	???	change 35% to a decimal and multiply (= 18.2)
(2) What percent of 52 is 18.2?	???	×	52	=	18.2	divide 18.2 by 52; change the resultant decimal to percent (.35 = 35%)
(3) 35% of what is 18.2?	35%	×	???	=	18.2	divide 18.2 by 0.35 to get 52

Practice Set VII - 6

Solve each of the following:

1) 5% of 1000

7) 20% of 555

2) 50% of 1000

8) 12.5% of 480

3) 6.25% of 800

4) 10% of 750

5) 25% of 1200

6) 16.67% of 180

9) 33.3% of 500

10) 20% of 500

11) 37.5% of 1200

12) 40% of 1200

Word problems are practical situations where various mathematical procedures are used. The following are examples of percentage word problems.

Example:

A clinic has 43,560 square feet of floor space. An expansion is planned that will increase the floor space 25%. (a.) Find the amount of floor space that is being added. (b) Find the total floor space after the addition.

$$\begin{array}{r} 43{,}560 \\ \underline{\times .25} \\ 10{,}890.00 \end{array}$$

floor space added: 10,890 sq. ft.

43,560 sq. ft. + 10,890 sq. ft. = 54, 450 sq. ft.

floor space + increased space = total floor space after addition

Practice Set VII - 7

Solve the following word problems:

1. One veterinarian figured a job at $940.00. A second bid 25% less. What was the second bid?

2. Seventy-five pounds of brass contains 45% zinc and the balance is copper. Determine the number of pounds of zinc.

3. A shipment of chemicals was billed at $548.00 but it was damaged in transit. An allowance of 15% was made for the damages. What is the net amount due?

4. A technician measured 500 ml of distilled water. Eighteen percent of the water was used in the lab. How much distilled water was left?

Determining what percent one number is of another

Example: 20 is what percent of 50 or written another way: 20 = ? % of 50

Write the numbers as a fraction. The number to be compared (20) is the numerator. The number with which it to be compared (50) is the denominator.

$\frac{20}{50} = \frac{2}{5}$ change the fraction to a decimal

$5\overline{)2.0}$ = .4 change 0.4 to percent

0.4 = 40% 20 is 40% of 50.

Example: In measuring 80 lbs. of chemicals, 1.6 pounds was lost by accident. What percent was lost?

1.6 = ? % of 80 thus, $\frac{1.6}{80}$ and $80\overline{)1.60}$ = .02 and .02 = 2% was lost

Practice Set VII - 8

Solve the following problems:

1. Given 27 lbs. chemicals, 8 lbs. were lost. What percent was lost?

2. Given 125 lbs. of chemicals, 2.56 lbs. was lost. What percent was lost?

3. Given 11 lbs. of chemicals, 1.1 lbs. was lost. What percent loss?

4. Inspecting 50 bottles from a box, 4 were found broken. What percent were broken?

5. In working 45 problems on a test, 7 were incorrect. What percent were incorrect?

6. After 11 days at work you missed one day. What percent have you missed? (12 days total)

7. A man working for \$6.40 per hour has his pay increased by 52 cents per hour. What percent increase did he receive?

8. John feeds his dogs 2 $^{3}/_{4}$ pounds of dog food from a canister containing 12 lbs. of food. What percent of the food was removed?

9. For a certain laboratory experiment, a resultant weighing 3.25 lbs. is obtained. If the total weight of the chemical components of the experiment were 4.59 lbs. , then the weight of the resultant is what percent of the components?

10. Cage raw materials weigh 327 lbs. Finished cages weigh 288 lbs. What percent of the raw material is lost in manufacture?

Finding a new price when there is a percent change is often necessary. This could be the result of a price increase due to inflation or a price decrease due to a discount. Either way, the procedures are similar.

Price Increase

1. Find the change by converting the percent to its decimal equivalent and multiplying by the price.
2. Add the increase in the price to the original price to find the new price.

Example: 9% increase in an object which originally cost $15.49

9% = 0.09 decimal equivalent

$$\begin{array}{l} \$15.49 \\ \underline{\times 0.09} \\ \$1.3941 = \$1.39 \end{array} \quad \text{price increase}$$

$$\begin{array}{l} \$15.49 \\ \underline{+\,1.39} \\ \$16.88 \end{array} \quad \text{new price}$$

Price Decrease

1. Find the change by converting the percent to its decimal equivalent and multiplying by the price.
2. Subtract the decrease in price from the original price to find the new price.

Example: 6% decrease in object which originally cost $8.95

6% = 0.06 decimal equivalent

$$\begin{array}{l} \$8.95 \\ \underline{\times\, 0.06} \\ \$0.537 = 54 \text{ cents} \end{array}$$

$$\begin{array}{rl} \$8.95 & \text{original price} \\ \underline{-\ .54} & \text{price decrease} \\ \$8.41 & \text{new price} \end{array}$$

Practice Set VII - 9 Find the new price (cost) for each of the following:

1) 6.6% increase on an original price of $5.47

2) 5% decrease on an original price of $10.

3) 2% decrease from an original price of $5.39

4) 8% increase from an original price of $3.35

5) 11% increase on an original price of $6.98

Practice Set VII - 10

1. Evaluate each of the following:

   a. 16% of 28

   b. 90% of 1,000

c. 10% of 1,600

d. 17% of 32

e. 11 $^{1}/_{2}$% of 980

f. 13% of 78

g. $^{1}/_{4}$% of 13

h. 7 $^{1}/_{4}$% of 100

2. The kennel area is to be enlarged by 25%. The present size is 1,230 square feet.

a. How much additional space will be available?

b. What will be the total area when complete?

Practice Set VII - 11

The following items are taken from two price lists. Company A gives a 22% discount, while Company B's prices have increased by 7 $^{1}/_{2}$%. Find the new prices of each company.

Item	Company A list price	Company A new price	Company B list price	Company B new price
general operating scissors	$6.10	________	$4.45	________
Metzenbaum scissors	$8.30	________	$6.25	________
iris scissors	$7.05	________	$5.00	________
Allis tissue forceps	$7.58	________	$5.55	________
surgical cotton wadding	2.00/dz	________	1.70/dz	________
Kelly forceps	$5.20	________	$3.52	________
Needle holders	$4.25	________	$3.00	________
Gauze sponges	60.00/cs	________	42.75/cs	________
Endotracheal tubes	$2.38	________	$1.93	________
First-aid dressing	4.80/dz	________	3.55/dz	________
Mayo intestinal needles	2.55/dz	________	1.75/dz	________

Solutions - General

The term *gram per deciliter* is used in hospital medicine, such as for hemoglobin determinations where the amount may be expressed as 14g/dl for example. Gram percent (g%) means parts per 100 ml. More recently, the term gram per deciliter has become popular. Both terms describe a ratio of mass per unit volume.

Example: 12 grams in 100 ml. of solution is termed 12 gram percent or 12 g%.

Note that 100 ml = 1 deciliter

$$\frac{12\,g}{100\,ml} = \frac{12\,g}{1\,dl}$$

Practice Set VII - 12 Express each of the following as grams percent or grams per 100 ml.

1) 14 g/100 ml =

2) 0.9 g/100 ml =

3) 0.5 g/100 ml =

4) 1 g/100 ml =

5) 18 g% =

6) 9 g% =

7) 0.003 g% =

8) 4.5 g% =

9) 0.85 g% =

10) 4 g/100 ml =

Sometimes the quantity is very small and the term milligram percent (mg%) is used. This means the number of mg per 100 ml.

Example: 5 mg in 100 ml of solution is termed 5 mg percent or 5mg%

Convert:

11.) 3.2 mg/100 ml =

12.) .4 mg/100 ml =

13.) 0.1 mg% =

14.) 17 mg% =

Practice Set VII - 13

1. The *packed cell volume* (PCV) in blood analysis is divided by 3 to obtain the amount of hemoglobin (Hbg). This is recorded in g/100 ml or gram percent or gram/deciliter. Calculate the following in g% (The weight of Hbg is measured in grams and the volume of blood in ml.)

Example: PCV was measured at 51. 51 ÷ 3 = 17; so Hbg is 17g% or 17 g / dl

	PCV	
a.	36	dog_1
b.	22	dog_2
c.	24	cat_1
d.	42	cat_2
e.	30	pig_1
f.	48	pig_2

2. Solutions whose concentration are given in % means grams (g) per 100 milliliters (ml) or milliliters per 100 milliliters if liquid. Calculate the concentration in % for each of the following.

a. 0.9 g of sodium chloride in 100 ml of solution

b. 5 g of dextrose in 100 ml of solution

c. 4.5 g of dextrose in 100 ml of solution

d. 10 ml of formalin in 100 ml of solution

e. 2 g of copper sulfate in 100 ml of solution

f. 1 g of copper sulfate in 100 ml of solution

g. 70 ml of isopropyl alcohol in 100 ml of solution

h. 2 ml of formalin in 100 ml of solution

i. 9 g of glucose in 100 ml of solution

3. Convert to decimal or %

a. 0.237

b. 2.37

c. 23.7

d. 237

e. 0.0237

f. 0.00237

g. 0.000237

h. 45%

i. 0.1%

j. 43.27%

k. 8.32%

l. 9.372%

m. 0.3271%

n. 0.16137%

Chapter 8

Ratio and Proportion

Objectives

Upon completion, the student must be able to do the following:

- **Express two quantities as a ratio and find its value.**
- **Express a ratio in lowest terms.**
- **Determine ratios from medical labels.**
- **Solve proportions.**

The study of ratios provides the background necessary to solve dosage problems involving ratio and proportion.

In a clinical lab it is often necessary to compare two (or more) things which are alike in some manner such as size, number, or weight. The comparison of one quantity with another like quantity is called a ratio. For example, suppose you compare a dime and a nickel. Both involve money, but are of different size and weight (among other differences.) We could compare their values and write a ratio as 10 cents to 5 cents. We could indicate this ratio as 10 : 5 using a colon to represent the ratio 10 to 5. Another way this ratio could be represented is as a fraction: $\frac{10}{5}$. All the rules governing fractions apply to ratios as well.

Here's another *example:*

Compare these two circles:

A

Diameter: 9

B

Diameter: 15

The diameter of circle A compared to the diameter of circle B may be written as the *ratio*:

9 to 15 or 9:15 or $\frac{9}{15}$

This last can be reduced: $\frac{9}{15} = \frac{3}{5}$ $\frac{3}{5}$ or 3 : 5

	First term		Second term
Notice that a ratio has two terms:	9	:	15

Practice Set VIII - 1

Read the following problems and express the information given as a ratio:

(a) If a graduated cylinder "A" has 80 milliliters of solution and a second graduated cylinder "B" has 40 milliliters of the solution, what is the ratio of "A" to "B"? [answer 80:40]

(b) Refer to the previous problem (a). What is the ratio of "B" to "A"?

(c) Two dogs, "A" and "B" are weighed separately. "A" weighs 60 pounds and "B" weighs 25 pounds. What is the (weight) ratio of "A" to "B"?

(d) A solution mixture has the ratio of one part hydrochloric acid (HCL), 70 parts Ethyl Alcohol (EtOH), and 29 parts water. What is the ratio of EtOH to water?

(e) In the preceding problem (d), what is the ratio of water to HCL?

The value of a ratio is found by dividing the numerator by the denominator.

Examples:

value

(a) 4:5 or $\frac{4}{5}$ ⟶ $\frac{4}{5} = 0.8$

(b) 3:6 or $\frac{3}{6}$ ⟶ $\frac{3}{6} = \frac{1}{2} = 0.5$

Ratios are always expressed in lowest terms (as are fractions).

Examples:

(a) 5:10 or $\frac{5}{10} = \frac{1}{2}$ or 1 : 2

(b) 3:9 or $\frac{3}{9} = \frac{1}{3}$ or 1 : 3

Practice Set VIII - 2

Convert each ratio to fraction form (reduce where necessary) and find the value of the ratio:

(a) 5 : 15 (b) 9 : 81 (c) 17 : 51

(d) 6 : 12 (e) 8 : 64 (f) 9 : 10

The value of a ratio does not change when both the numerator and denominator are multiplied (or divided) by the same number. (Exactly as with fractions.)

Examples:

(a) $\frac{1}{2} \times \frac{3}{3} = \frac{3}{6}$ (b) $\frac{3 \div 3}{6 \div 3} = \frac{1}{2}$

Ratios usually have the same units.

Examples:

(a) 10 feet : 40 feet (b) 1 cc : 50 cc (c) 4 in : 40 in

However, in clinical laboratory conditions, sometimes have dissimilar units.

Examples:

(a) 5 mg : 1 cc

$$\frac{5mg}{1cc}$$

(b) 1 cc : 5 lb. body wt.

$$\frac{1cc}{5lbs}$$

Practice Set VIII - 3

Write the ratios for the following. Be sure to include units. (Note: This is a first step in solving dosage problems.)

(a) There are 5 grams of surital found in 100 ml of solution.

(b) There are 10 mg of sodium caparsolate in every 1 ml of solution.

(c) There are 100 mg of Thiamine in every 1 cc of solution.

(d) The dosage for Vitamin B complex is 1 ml for every 100 lbs body weight.

(e) Thorazine contains 25 mg in every ml.

(f) 0.1 mg of Thorazine is given for every 2.0 kg of body weight.

(g) 1 cc of sodium pentobarbital is given for every 5 lb of body weight.

Medicine bottles and labels

Working in a clinic or lab may involve using the information from a medicine bottle label to determine dosage. It is your responsibility to determine the correct dosage even if the unit dosage is provided.

A lot of information is provided on the medicine bottle label itself and / or the package insert. Your understanding and comprehension of dosage and concentration and their meanings cannot be minimized.

You will be given the opportunity to learn and practice reading and interpreting the information commonly available on dosage and concentration.

Dosage is generally provided in terms of how much to administer per pound, kilogram, or individual animal.

Examples:

$\frac{5mg}{10lbs}$ $\frac{1cc}{5lbs}$ 1 capsule per individual $\frac{1cc}{1kg}$

When dosage is provided per individual it is usually stated as the number of capsules, tablets, cc, mg, or so forth to be administered.

Concentration is expressed in terms of how much per unit of medication.

Examples:

$$\frac{5\ mg}{\text{tablet}} \qquad \frac{250\ mg}{\text{capsule}} \qquad \frac{1000\ mg}{1\text{cc}}$$

Most dosage problems can be solved using proportions. A proportion is composed of two ratios that are equal. The ratios 1 : 2 and 12 : 24 form a proportion since the two ratios are equal. A proportion can be written 1 : 2 = 12 : 24 which is read " 1 is to 2 as 12 is to 24." A proportion is more commonly written as $\frac{1}{2} = \frac{12}{24}$. Typically, three of the values are known and there is an unknown fourth value.

$$\frac{①}{②} = \frac{③}{④}$$

Like this

$$\frac{7}{21} = \frac{?}{3}$$

The parts of a proportion: If we had two ratios such as 1 : 3 and 4 : 12 which represent equal quantities, they can be expressed as a proportion one way as ...

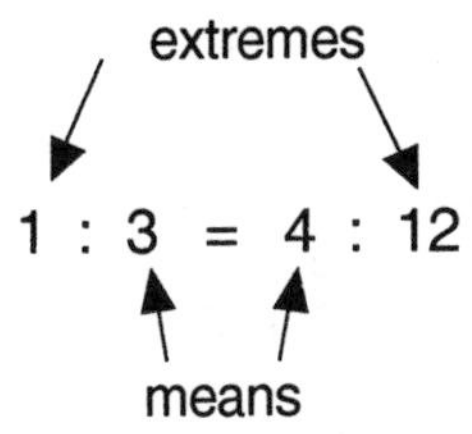

extremes

1 : 3 = 4 : 12

means

The two outside terms (1 and 12) are called extremes. The two inner terms (3 and 4) are called means. In any proportion, the product of the extremes equals the product of the means. Try it!

Another way to express a proportion is in fraction form [this is the preferred method]:

Example:

1 : 3 = 4 : 12 can be written $\frac{1}{3} = \frac{4}{12}$

When written in this manner, a missing, or unknown, element of the proportion can be determined by cross-multiplying.

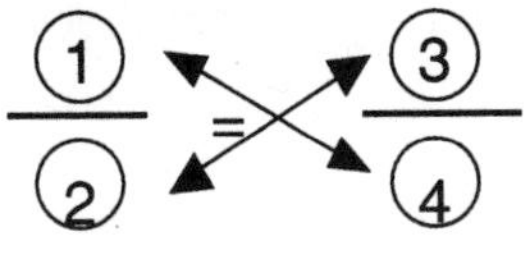

$$\frac{①}{②} = \frac{③}{④}$$

Example:

2 : 5 = 8 : n or $\frac{2}{5} = \frac{8}{n}$ n represents the unknown term

cross-multiply: 2 x n = 2n and 5 x 8 = 40

yields the equation: 2n = 40

In order to solve this equation, the 2 must be eliminated from the left-hand side of the equation. Since 2n indicates multiplication, undo that by using division. Divide each side of the equation by 2.

$$\frac{\cancel{2}n}{\cancel{2}} = \frac{40}{2}$$ dividing both sides of the equation by 2 and canceling the twos on the left-hand side

$$n = 20$$

Check for the correct solution by multiplying the means and the extremes: $2 \times 20 = 5 \times 8$!

Some helpful rules governing proportions:

Both sides of the proportion equality can be:

- multiplied by the same number without changing the value of the proportion.
- divided by the same number without changing the value of the proportion.
- added to by the same number without changing the value of the proportion.
- subtracted to or from by the same number without changing its value.
- inverted without changing its value.

Tip: to solve a proportion by cross-multiplication, multiply the two numbers diagonally opposite each other and divide by the number that is diagonally opposite the unknown.

Examples:

(a) $\frac{12}{③} = \frac{n}{4}$ multiply the two numbers diagonally opposite

divide by the number diagonally opposite the unknown (here it's 3)

$$n = (12 \times 4) \div 3$$

$$n = 48 \div 3$$

$$n = 16$$

(b) $\frac{n}{7} = \frac{10}{35}$ multiply diagonally across the equals sign; divide by the 35 since 35 has no number to multiply by

$n = \frac{7 \times 10}{35}$

$n = 2$

(c) $\frac{5}{n} = \frac{35}{56}$

$n = \frac{5 \times 56}{35}$

$n = 8$

Practice Set VIII - 4

Find the value of the unknown term in each of the following proportions:

(a) $n{:}200 = 1{:}10$

(b) $1{:}15 = 0.2{:}n$

(c) $1{:}15 = 0.1{:}x$

(d) $\frac{x}{2000} = \frac{.85}{100}$

(e) $\frac{1/6}{1/8} = \frac{x}{30}$

(f) $\frac{3}{6} = \frac{1}{x}$

(g) $\frac{1}{5000} = \frac{.2}{a}$

(h) $\frac{2}{n} = \frac{22}{33}$

(i) $\frac{0.9}{100} = \frac{x}{1000}$

(j) $\frac{14}{n} = \frac{7}{28}$

(k) $\frac{10}{100} = \frac{x}{4}$

(l) $\frac{x}{16} = \frac{8}{64}$

(m) $5:100 = 20:x$

(n) $\frac{14}{12} = \frac{7}{x}$

(o) $\frac{1}{50} = \frac{x}{1/2}$

Problems found in a clinical setting usually have units associated with them. When solving these problems, make certain to include the units. Units, by the way, will "cancel" just as numbers did when multiplying and dividing fractions and the same rules apply.

Note: since the letter "x" is frequently used to signify, or stand in for, an unknown quantity, we will use the more conventional "dot or an asterisk (*)" to signify multiplication.

Example:

$$\frac{x}{5lbs} = \frac{2mg}{10lbs}$$ cross-multiply as usual

$$x = \frac{2mg \cdot 5\cancel{lbs}}{10\cancel{lbs}}$$ the pounds units cancel

$$x = \frac{2mg \cdot \cancel{5}^{1}}{\cancel{10}_{2}}$$ numbers cancel as usual

$$x = \frac{\cancel{2}mg}{\cancel{2}}$$ continue canceling; remember $\frac{2}{2} = 1$

$$x = 1mg$$

The units can also be used to check the result. If the answer had been in pounds, there would have been some type of error somewhere.

Practice Set VIII - 5

Solve the following proportions. Be sure your answer includes the proper units.

(a) $\frac{300mg}{x} = \frac{10mg}{1ml}$

(b) $\frac{2lbs}{4cc} = \frac{10lbs}{x}$

(c) $\frac{x}{10lbs} = \frac{1cc}{25lbs}$

(d) $\frac{x}{1400lbs} = \frac{5mg}{100lbs}$

Practice Set VIII - 6

Solve the following:

(a) $\frac{x}{2} = \frac{3}{6}$

(b) $\frac{x}{8} = \frac{10}{16}$

(c) $\frac{x}{17} = \frac{3}{51}$

(d) $\frac{x}{9} = \frac{21}{24}$

(e) $\frac{x}{6} = \frac{3}{16}$

(f) $\frac{x}{7} = \frac{5}{9}$

(g) $\frac{x}{3} = \frac{9}{1}$

(h) $\frac{x}{2.5} = \frac{8}{3}$

(i) $\frac{8}{x} = \frac{16}{3}$

(j) $\frac{4}{x} = \frac{7}{11}$

(k) $\frac{3}{4} = \frac{75}{x}$

(l) $\frac{2.5}{6} = \frac{x}{25}$

(m) $\frac{13}{14} = \frac{10}{x}$

(n) $\frac{12}{30} = \frac{x}{5}$

(o) $\frac{13}{39} = \frac{9}{x}$

(p) $\frac{14}{28} = \frac{x}{8.5}$

(q) $\frac{3}{9} = \frac{5}{x}$

(r) $\frac{1.8mg}{1cc} = \frac{3.5mg}{x}$

(s) $\frac{1cc}{5lbs} = \frac{x}{35lbs}$

(t) $\frac{1cc}{10lbs} = \frac{x}{35lbs}$

(u) $\frac{1cc}{5lbs} = \frac{x}{65lbs}$

Chapter 8 Review

Solve each of the following. Be sure to show units where applicable. Round answers to 3 decimal places, if applicable. Reduce to lowest terms.

(a) $\frac{x}{7.5lbs} = \frac{0.25mg}{1lb}$

(b) $\frac{1drop}{5cc} = \frac{n}{35cc}$

(c) $\frac{10mg}{1ml} = \frac{70mg}{x}$

(d) $\frac{55mg}{n} = \frac{10mg}{1ml}$

(e) $\frac{0.5mg}{1cc} = \frac{7.5mg}{a}$

(f) $\frac{1cc}{25lbs} = \frac{a}{58lbs}$

(g) $\frac{x}{500ml} = \frac{4g}{100ml}$

(h) $\frac{a}{1000ml} = \frac{0.9g}{100ml}$

(i) $\frac{160mg}{n} = \frac{40mg}{1cc}$

(j) $\frac{x}{17lbs} = \frac{1mg}{1lb}$

(k) $\frac{x}{30cc} = \frac{1drop}{5cc}$

(l) $\frac{x}{5.5lbs} = \frac{0.5mg}{1lb}$

(m) $\frac{x}{5.5lbs} = \frac{0.25mg}{1lb}$

(n) $\frac{x}{800ml} = \frac{2.5g}{100ml}$

(o) $\frac{160mg}{x} = \frac{20mg}{1cc}$

(p) $\frac{180mg}{x} = \frac{6mg}{10cc}$

(q) $\frac{x}{25lbs} = \frac{\frac{1}{4}mg}{1lb}$

(r) $\frac{x}{24cc} = \frac{1drop}{5cc}$

(s) $\frac{325mg}{x} = \frac{25mg}{1ml}$

(t) $\frac{x}{14lb} = \frac{0.25mg}{1lb}$

(u) $\frac{20mg}{1cc} = \frac{3.50mg}{x}$

(v) $\frac{x}{1600lbs} = \frac{2mg}{100lbs}$

(w) $\frac{32mg}{x} = \frac{10mg}{1ml}$

(x) $\frac{x}{1250lbs} = \frac{4mg}{100lbs}$

(y) $\frac{x}{2000lbs} = \frac{3mg}{100lbs}$

(z) $\frac{n}{25lbs} = \frac{1cc}{5lbs}$

(aa) $\frac{5mg}{n} = \frac{6mg}{1ml}$

(bb) $\frac{13mg}{x} = \frac{25mg}{1ml}$

(cc) $\frac{n}{7.5lbs} = \frac{0.1mg}{1lb}$

(dd) $\frac{18mg}{x} = \frac{20mg}{1ml}$

(ee) $\frac{0.5mg}{1lb} = \frac{x}{8.5lbs}$

(ff) $\frac{x}{9lbs} = \frac{1cc}{25lbs}$

(gg) $\frac{x}{13lbs} = \frac{\frac{1}{4}mg}{1lb}$

(hh) $\frac{n}{21lbs} = \frac{1cc}{5lbs}$

(ii) $\frac{23mg}{x} = \frac{40mg}{1cc}$

(jj) $\frac{2.4mg}{x} = \frac{6mg}{1ml}$

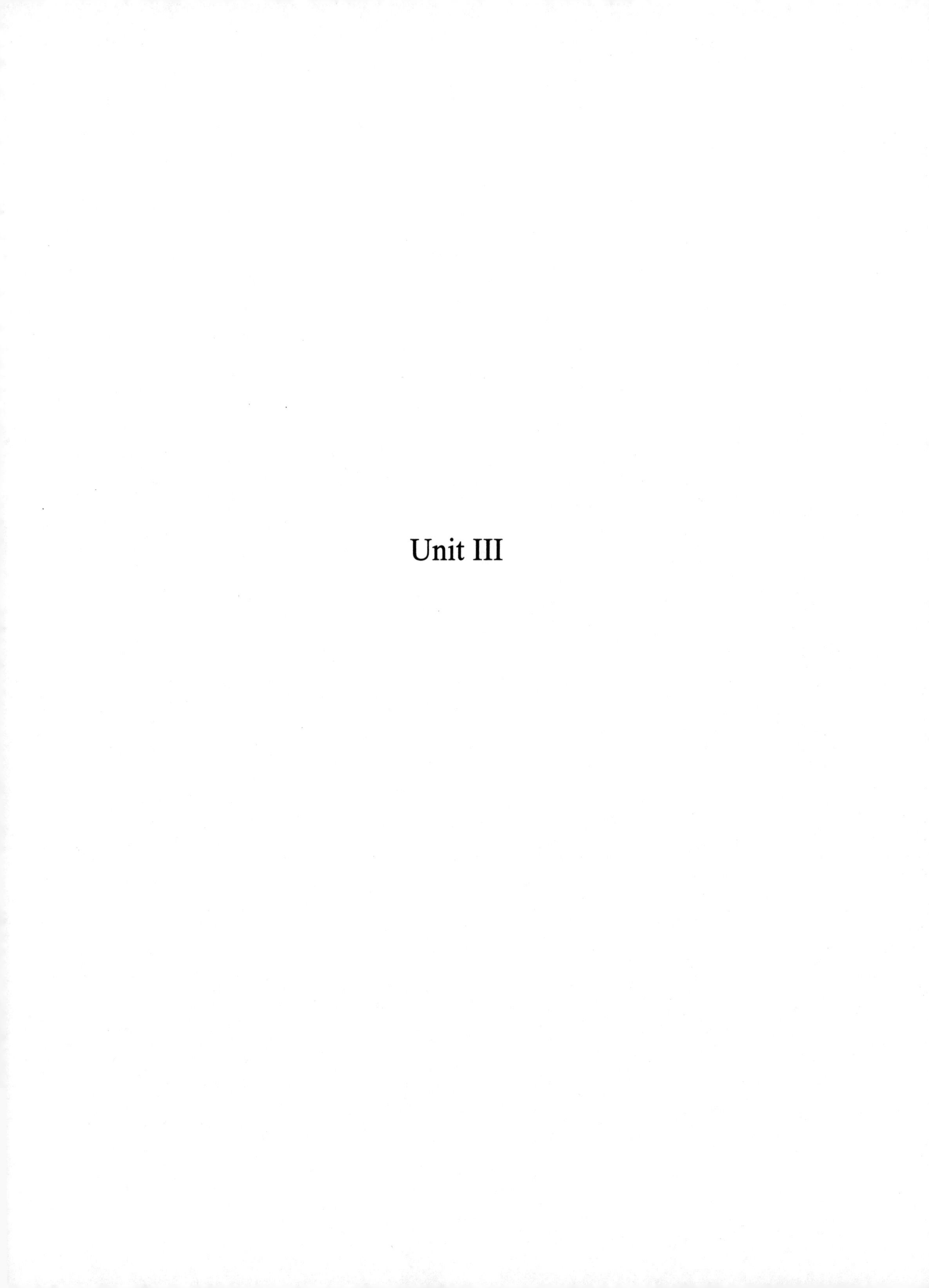

Unit III

Chapter 9

Dosage and Concentration Applications

Using Ratios and Proportions

Objectives

Upon completion, the student must be able to do the following:

- **model and solve dosage and concentration problems.**
- **model and solve multiple-step problems.**

Understanding and solving word problems involves some of the most critical skills a technician can learn. After all, we communicate both orally and with the written word. This is how we work together in an office or clinic. The doctor who asks for 3 cc of atropine for an injection, for instance, trusts the technician to supply exactly that. The calculation of dosages is a critical area — it must be done quickly and accurately.

When solving word problems, there are several principles that are useful:

- Decide what is being asked. What is needed for the result?
- Catalog the information given – write it down!
- Determine the ratio and proportions including what is unknown and the units.

Example:

A dose of sodium pentobarbital is needed for a 125 pound dog. The dosage given on the label is 1 cc per 5 pounds of body weight.

1. What is needed? - the amount to administer to the dog is "x" cc.

2. Known information: dosage of $\frac{1cc}{5lbs}$ and weight of dog - 125 pounds.

3. Determine the appropriate proportion: $\frac{Xcc}{125lbs} = \frac{1cc}{5lbs}$

4. Solve:

$$\frac{Xcc}{125lbs} = \frac{1cc}{5lbs}$$

the lbs units cancel; 5 divides evenly into 125

$$Xcc = \frac{\overset{25}{\cancel{125}}\cancel{lbs} \times 1cc}{\underset{1}{\cancel{5}}\cancel{lbs}}$$

$$X = 25cc$$

The correct dosage for the 125 pound dog is 25 cc.

Practice Set IX - 1

Solve the following problems:

(a) How much Surital is needed for a dog weighing 25 pounds? Dosage is 1 cc per 5 lbs.

(b) How much Surital would be necessary if the dog weighed 67 pounds?

(c) A tranquilizer, Nortron, is used at the rate of 4 mg per 1 pound of body weight. How much is needed for a 40 pound dog?

(d) Each tablet of Nortron contains 10 mg. What is the nearest whole number of tablets necessary for the dog in (c)?

(e) How much ketomine is necessary for a 10 pound cat? Dosage is 15 mg per 1 lb.

(f) Since the amount of ketomine needed has been determined in (e); calculate the number of cc necessary if the concentration is 100 mg per 1 cc.

(g) A solution consists of 10 g of NaOH in 100 ml of solution. Determine the amount of NaOH in 200 ml of a solution of the same concentration.

(h) 100 ml of a solution containing 0.5 g Methylene Blue and 1 ml of Formalin (with a total volume of 100 ml). How much Methylene Blue would be needed to make 1200 ml of solution of the same concentration?

(i) A solution is to be made using 1 g of Giemsa in 50 ml of solution. How much of the Giemsa will be needed to make 3000 ml of that solution?

(j) The veterinarian needs a solution containing 0.3 g Wrights and 0.03 g Giemsa in 100 ml of solution. How much of each of those chemicals will be needed to make 3000 ml of the solution.

(k) You are making a solution which calls for 0.6 g NaCl, 0.03 g KCl, 2.02 g $CaCl_2$, and 0.31 g sodium lactate in 100 ml of solution. If 5000 ml of solution is needed, how much of each of the components will you add?

(l) If 9 dogs cages cost $450, how many cages can be purchased for $1000 ?

(m) If 8 dog feeders cost $72, how much will 19 dog feeders cost?

(n) If a 10 lb dog requires 2.5 cc of medication, how many cc will a 25 lb dog require?

Some medicines in the veterinary clinic are prescribed in milligrams per pound of body weight, yet they're packaged in milligrams per cc. To compute the proper dosage requires multiple steps:

- calculate the number of mg to be given for a particular weight of animal
- calculate the number of cc which contains the number of mg computed

Example: Ketomine is given at the dosage of 15 mg per 1 lb body weight. It is packaged in the bottle at a concentration of 100 mg per 1 cc. How many cc should be given to a 27 lb cat?

1. Determine the amount of ketomine in mg based upon the 27 lb cat.

$$\frac{x}{27lbs} = \frac{15mg}{1lbs}$$ cross-multiply and simplify

$$x = \frac{27lbs \times 15mg}{1lbs}$$

$$x = 405mg$$

2. This gives the amount of medicine necessary. Determine the cc equivalent.

$$\frac{405mg}{x} = \frac{100mg}{1cc}$$ solve the proportion by cross-multiplying and simplifying

$$x = \frac{405mg \times 1cc}{100mg}$$

$$x = 4.05cc$$

Practice Set IX - 2

(a) How many cc of ketomine should be administered to a 17 pound cat when the doctor has prescribed a dosage of 15 mg per pound of body weight? The ketomine is packaged in a concentration of 100 mg per 1 cc.

(b) Phenobarbitol is given to a dog at the rate of 3mg per pound of body weight. The dog weighs 42 pounds. The concentration is 50 mg per cc. How many cc should be administered?

(c) Prednisaolone is prescribed in a dosage of 0.5 mg / lb. for a 15 pound dog. How many cc are necessary if the concentration is 5 mg per cc?

(d) Sulfamethazine is to be given to a 30 pound dog at the rate of 25 mg / lb. How many cc are necessary if the concentration is 10 mg per cc?

(e) Morphine has been prescribed at the rate of 2 mg / lb for a 125 pound dog. The concentration is 15 mg per cc. How many cc should be administered?

Solutions that are prepared from concentrations can be made by determining the value of the percent of concentration and changing this to grams. Dissolve the appropriate gram amount in water to make 100 ml of the correct concentration of the needed solution.

Review of terms

% means parts per 100

grams% means grams per 100 ml

Thus, the term % can represent either grams per 100 ml or ml per 100 ml

Example:

A 0.9% sodium chloride solution is required. Use 0.9 grams of sodium chloride and dissolve this in water to make 100 ml of solution.

The problem can be more complex if the desired volume is not 100 ml. For example, how much sodium chloride would be needed to prepare only 60 ml of solution?

Solve this problem using the same ratio and proportion methods you have been using.

It is known that: $\frac{0.9g}{100ml}$ but what is needed is $\frac{?g}{60ml}$ in order to achieve the correct concentration.

$$\frac{x}{60ml} = \frac{0.9g}{100ml}$$

cross-multiply and simplify. The ml units cancel

$$x = \frac{0.9g \times 60\cancel{ml}}{100\cancel{ml}}$$

$$x = 0.54g$$

Thus, 0.54 grams of sodium chloride is needed to make 60 ml of 0.9% solution.

Example:

A solution is composed of 95 ml of water and 5 ml of formalin. Determine the amount of formalin necessary to make 1000 ml of solution of the same concentration.

Total volume of known solution: 95 ml + 5 ml = 100 ml

For every 100 ml of solution, 5 ml of formalin is needed. Writing as a proportion:

$$\frac{5ml}{100ml} = \frac{x}{1000ml}$$

$$x = \frac{5ml \times 1000ml}{100ml}$$

$$x = 50ml$$

So, 50 ml of formalin is needed to make 1000 ml of the formalin solution.

Practice Set IX - 3

(a) Prepare 4000 ml of solution at 9% saline. How many grams of sodium chloride will be needed?

(b) Prepare 4000 ml solution of 5% dextrose.

(c) Prepare 1000 ml of 2.5% dextrose.

(d) Prepare a 500 ml solution of 10% dextrose.

(e) Prepare a 3000 ml solution of 5% formalin. (Formalin is measured in ml)

(f) Prepare 4000 ml of a solution of 10% formalin.

(g) Calculate the amount of each chemical needed to make 600 ml of the following solutions:

1. One (1) gram of Iodine in 100 ml of solution.

2. Two (2) g potassium Iodine in 100 ml of solution.

(h) If a solution calls for 2 ml Acetic Acid and 98 ml of H_2O, and if 1600 ml of the solution is needed; How much acetic acid should be used?

(i) If 1000 ml of a certain solution contains 1.5 g NaCl, How many grams of NaCl are needed to make 1500 ml of the solution?

(j) It takes 1 g of mercuric bichloride to make 1000 ml of solution. How many grams of mercuric bichloride would it take to make 750 ml of solution?

(k) In making a 2% solution, 10 g of boric acid crystals are dissolved in 500 ml of water. How many grams of boric acid crystals are needed to make 50 ml of solution?

(l) To prepare a certain solution, 1 g of potassium permanganate crystals is added to 5000 ml of water. How many grams of potassium permanganate crystals should be added to 2000 ml of water to make a similar concentration of the solution?

Practice Set IX - 4

Solve the following using ratio and proportion techniques. (B.W. = body weight)

(a) Surital can be used as an anesthetic in a dosage of 1 cc per 5 lbs B.W. How much should be used in each of the following cases:

(i) For a 15 lb cat? (ii) For a 65 lb Boxer?

(b) Surital can also be used as an anesthetic in a dosage of 1 cc per 3 lbs B.W. How much should be used for each of the animals in (a) i and ii?

(c) To reduce salivation when using Surital, atropine can be used in a dosage of 1 cc per 25 lb B.W. How much should be used for each of the animals in (a) i and ii?

(d) Ketomine can be used an an intramuscular anesthetic for cats. The dosage is 15 mg per pound of B.W.

(i) How much should be administered to a 12 pound cat?

(ii) The ketomine comes dissolved in a liquid at 100 mg per cc. How many cc must be given for the prescribed dosage in part (i)?

(e) Amphesol (5%) is given as a stimulant at a dosage of 0.4 ml per 10 lbs B.W. How much is needed to stimulate a 35 pound dog?

(f) A tranquilizer, Nortran, is given to animals at the dosage of $^1/_4$ mg per lb B.W.

(i) How many mg will be needed for a female dog of 45 pounds in order to catherize her?

(ii) The Nortran is packaged in tablets of 10 mg each. Determine the nearest whole number of tablets needed for (i)

(g) A different tranquilizer, Jenoton, is administered at the rate of 1.5 mg per lb of B.W.

(i) How much is required for a 125 lb dog?

(ii) If the medication is packaged as a 25 mg per cc concentration, how many cc are needed?

(h) The number of WBC (white blood cells) can be estimated using viscosity measurements. Assuming a linear relationship, what is the estimated WBC count when the average flow time is 5 seconds if a 5000 WBC has an average flow time of 6 seconds?

(i) A boxer weighing 53 pounds has hook worms. DNP (45 mg/ml) is prescribed at the rate of 0.1 cc per lb of B.W. How much should be administered?

Practice Set IX - 5

(a) A dog weighing 35 pounds needs atropine sulfate ($^1/_{120}$ grain per cc) at the rate of 1 cc per 25 lbs B.W. How many cc are needed?

(b) Surital (5%) can be used as an anesthetic at a dosage of 1 cc per 5 lbs B.W. How many cc are needed for each of the following:

(i) 6 lb cat? (ii) 9 lb cat? (iii) 73 lb dog?

(iv) 35 lb dog? (v) 18 lb dog?

(c) Surital (5%) used as an anesthetic is packaged in solution 1 cc per 3 lbs B.W. How many cc are needed for each of the animals in (b)?

(d) Ketomine is an intramuscular anesthetic for cats at a dosage of 15 mg per lb B.W. The ketomine is dissolved in a liquid at 100 mg per cc. How many cc are needed for each of the following cats:

(i) 6 lb (ii) 8.5 lb (iii) 18 lb (iv) 13 lb (v) 45 lb

(e) A tranquilizer, Nortran, is used at the rate of $^1/_4$ mg per lb of B.W. Determine the amount necessary for each of the following dogs:

(i) 36 lb (ii) 125 lb (iii) 25 lb (iv) 73 lb (v) 18 lb

(f) The tranquilizer, Jenoton, is used at a rate of 1.5 mg per lb B.W. How much would be needed for each of the animals in (e)?

(g) DNP used for hookworms is prescribed at 0.1 cc per lb B.W. What is the dosage for each of the animals in (e)?

Practice Set IX - 6

(a) Pentobarbital is administered to a dog which weighs 35 pounds. The dosage rate is 1 cc per 5 lb B.W. (i) What is the total amount to be administered?

(ii) Only 60% is to be given immediately. How many cc will this be?

(iii) Shown is a 12 cc syringe. Assume that the syringe is filled with the amount calculated in (i). Indicate by an arrow (↓) on the syringe where this would be.

Indicate using a double arrow (↓↓) the point where the medication would be discharged to administer the initial 60%.

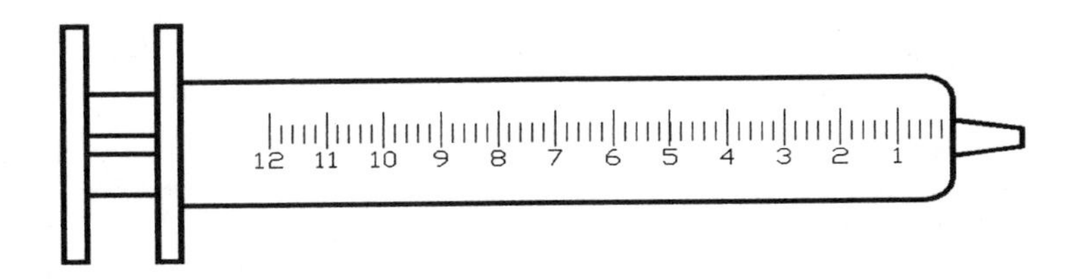

(b) Pentobarbital is to be administered to a 47 pound dog. The dosage is 1 cc per 5 lb.
(i) What is the total amount needed?

(ii) If 60% is administered initially, How many cc are needed?

(iii) Shown is a 12 cc syringe. Assume that the syringe is filled with the amount calculated in (i). Indicate by an arrow (↓) on the syringe where this would be.

Indicate using a double arrow (↓↓) the point where the medication would be discharged to administer the initial 60%.

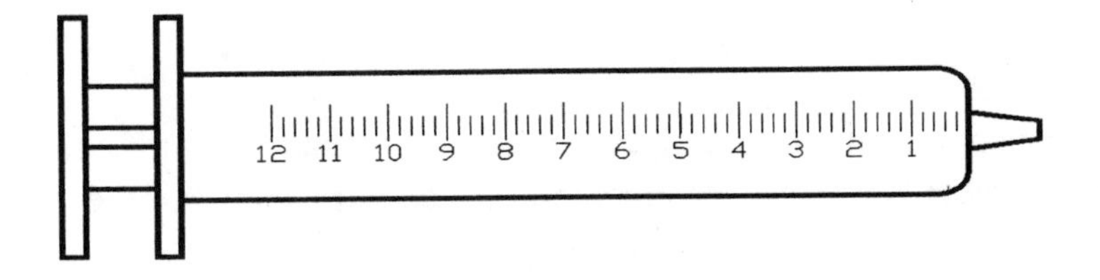

(c) Pentobarbital is prescribed for a dog which weighs 15 lbs. The dosage is 1 cc per 5 lb.

(i) What is the total amount of the prescribed dose?

(ii) 60% is to be administered initially. How many cc will that take?

(iii) Shown is a 12 cc syringe. Assume that the syringe is filled with the amount calculated in (i). Indicate by an arrow (↓) on the syringe where this would be. Indicate using a double arrow (↓↓) the point where the medication would be discharged to administer the initial 60%.

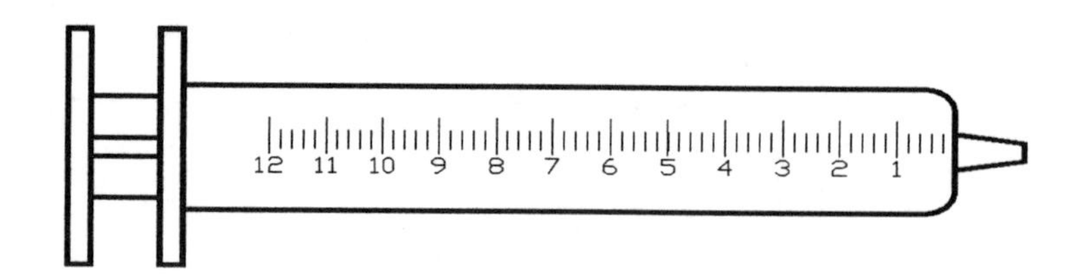

Practice Set IX - 7

1. For each of the following solutions, determine the number of grams (or ml if liquid) are necessary to:

(a) Make a 2500 ml solution of saline 0.9%

(b) Prepare a 525 ml solution of 2% formalin (consider the stock solution of 100% formalin and remember to use ml instead of grams since formalin is a liquid.)

(c) Prepare a 650 ml solution of 5% formalin.

(d) Prepare 950 ml of 5% dextrose solution.

(e) Make 3250 ml of 10% formalin solution.

(f) Make 75 ml of NaCl at 0.9%

(g) Prepare 25 ml of 1% alcoholic (in alcohol) solution of phenolphthalein.

(h) Make 95 ml of 1% $CuSO_4$.

(i) Make 200 ml of 10% Potassium Thiocyanate.

(j) Prepare 75 ml of a 1% silver nitrate solution.

(k) Prepare 35 ml of 1% $HgCl_2$ solution.

2. Calculate the percentage of solution for each of the following:

(a) 190 ml of ethyl alcohol in 200 ml of solution.

(b) 3.6 g of sodium chloride in 400 ml of water.

(c) 4.5 g of copper sulfate in 225 ml of solution.

(d) 15 g of glucose in 300 ml of solution.

(e) 4.5 g of sodium chloride in 500 ml of solution.

(f) 27 g of sodium chloride in 900 ml of solution.

(g) 210 ml of isopropyl alcohol in 300 ml of solution.

Practice Set IX - 8

(1) Surital can be used as a pre-anesthetic at a dosage of 1 cc per 5 lbs B.W. How much should you use for a 19 lb dog?

(2) Surital can also be used as an anesthetic at a dosage of 1 cc per 3 lb B.W. How much should you use for a 25 lb cat?

(3) To reduce salivation when using Surital, atropine can be used at a dosage of 1 cc per 20 lb B.W. How much should be used for a 9 lb cat?

(4) Ketomine can be used as an intramuscular anesthetic for cats. The dosage is 15 mg per lb of B.W. The ketomine is available in bottled form with a concentration of 100 mg per cc. How many cc are needed for a 14 lb cat?

(5) Amphesol (amphetamine sulfate) is given as a stimulant at a dosage of 0.4 ml per 10 lb B.W. How much is needed to stimulate a 30 pound dog?

(6) Nortran is given to animals at the dosage of $1/4$ mg per 1 lb B.W. (a) How much is needed for a 39 lb dog? (b) Notran comes in tablet form of 10 mg each. What is the nearest whole number of tablets necessary?

(7) Jenoton is given at the rate of 1.5 mg per lb B.W. to a 25 lb dog. It is packaged in a 25 mg per 1 cc concentration. How many cc are necessary for the dog?

(8) DNP used for hookworms is given at 0.1 cc per lb B.W. How much should be prescribed for a 75 lb dog?

(9) Prednisolone is prescribed for a 20 lb dog. The dosage is 0.5 mg per lb and the concentration is 5 mg per cc. How many cc are needed?

(10) Morphine has been prescribed at the rate of 2 mg per lb for a 93 lb dog. The concentration is 15 mg per cc. How many cc should you prepare?

(11) Make a 2000 ml solution of Normal saline 0.9%. How much salt (in grams) will you need to use?

(12) To prepare a 590 ml solution of 5% dextrose, how many grams of dextrose would you need?

(13) Prepare 85 ml of 0.9% saline. How much NaCl is needed?

(14) Make 50 ml of 1% alcoholic solution of phenolphthalein.

(15) Prepare 95 ml of 1% $CuSO_4$ solution. How many grams of $CuSO_4$ do you need?

(16) Ketomine is used for a 13 lb cat at 15 mg per lb. How many cc are needed if the concentration is 100 mg per cc?

(17) Surital is to be given to a 52 lb dog. The dosage is 1 cc per 5 lb. How many cc should you prepare?

(18) Phenobarbital is to be administered to a 24 lb dog at the rate of 2 cc / 5 lbs. How much do you need?

(19) Morphine is prescribed at 2 mg per lb; the concentration is 15 mg / cc. How many cc do you prepare for a 100 lb dog?

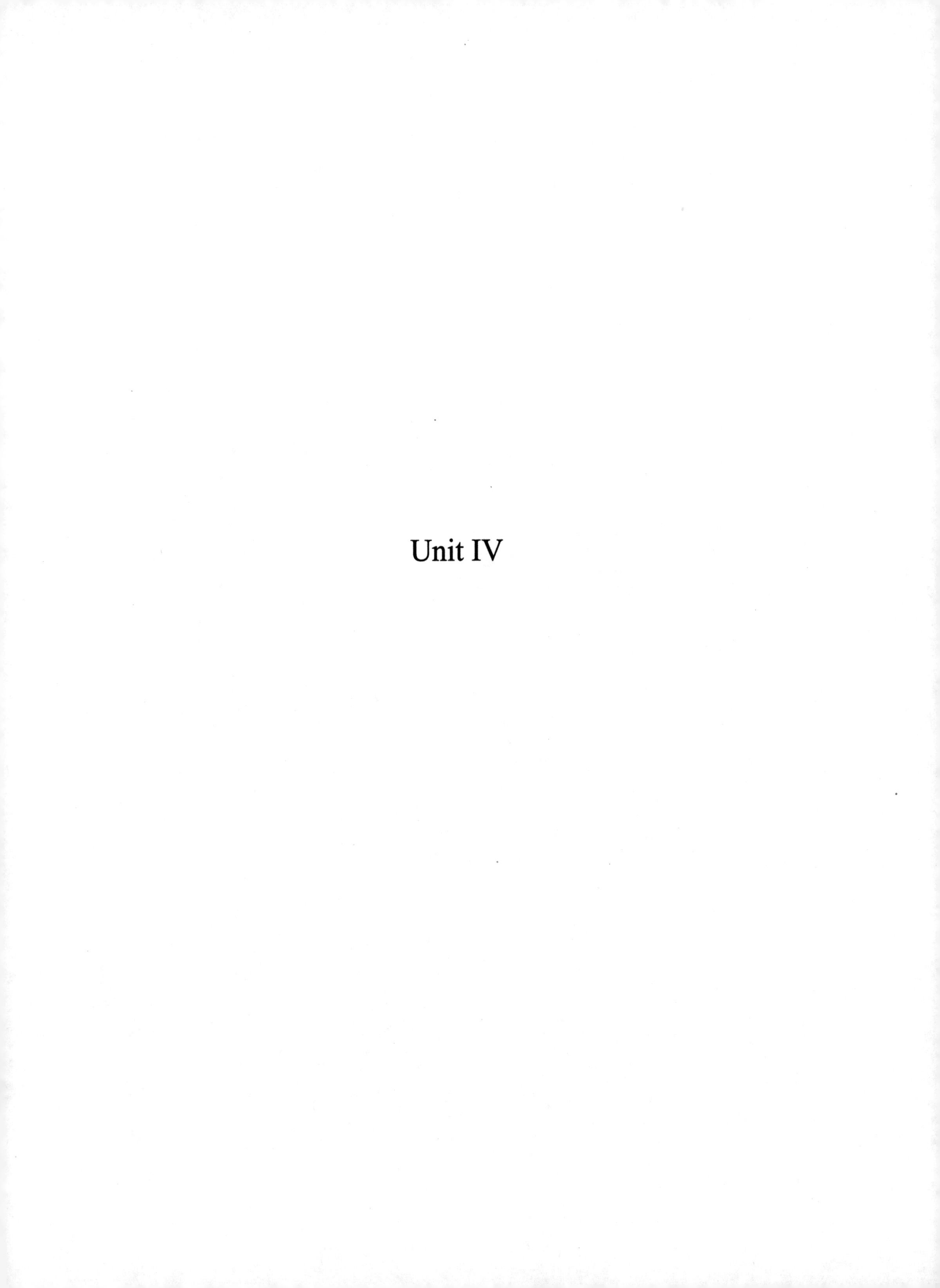

Unit IV

Chapter 10

The Metric System

Objectives

Upon completion, the student must be able to do the following:

- **List the prefixes and abbreviations used in the metric system.**
- **Convert metric quantities from larger to smaller units and vice versa.**
- **Be able to convert units using ratio and proportion techniques.**
- **Be able to convert using conversion factors.**

The metric system of measurement is the most widely used system in the world. It is a decimal system based upon powers of ten. The basic units of measurement are the meter for length, the liter for volume, and the gram for mass (weight). Multiples and fractional parts are formed by adding a prefix to the basic unit. The prefixes most commonly used are presented here. The prefixes as well as their meanings must be learned.

Decimal System	Numerical meaning	Metric Prefix	Abbreviation
Million	1,000,000	Mega-	M
Thousand	1,000	kilo-	k
Hundred	100	hecto-	h
Ten	10	deka-	dk
Unit	1	None	None
Tenth	0.1	deci-	d
Hundredth	0.01	centi-	c
Thousandth	0.001	milli-	m
Millionth	0.000001	micro-	μ
Billionth	0.000000001	nano-	n
Trillionth	1×10^{-12}	pico-	p

Practice Set X - 1

Write the appropriate metric prefix:

(a) hundreds ___________

(b) Tenths ___________

(c) Units ___________

(d) Thousands ___________

(e) Thousandths ___________

(f) Tens ___________

(g) Hundredths ___________

Common abbreviations along with the words for mass, length and volume are given in the chart below. A special note: the abbreviation for deka- has changed several times over the years. The student should be aware that s/he may encounter such variations as decameter (dam), decagram (dag) and decaliter (dal).

Prefix	Length	Weight	Volume
kilo-	kilometer (km)	kilogram (kg)	kiloliter (kl)
hecto-	hectometer (hm)	hectogram (hg)	hectoliter (hl)
deka-	dekameter (dkm)	dekagram (dkg)	dekaliter (dkl)
basic unit	meter (m)	gram (g)	liter (l)
deci-	decimeter (dm)	decigram (dg)	deciliter (dl)
centi-	centimeter (cm)	centigram (cg)	centiliter (cl)
milli-	millimeter (mm)	milligram (mg)	milliliter (ml)
micro-	micrometer (μm)	microgram (μg)	microliter (μl)

The line drawing from chapter 6 is reproduced here. The ability to recreate this chart on demand will prove to be an invaluable aid in mastering this material.

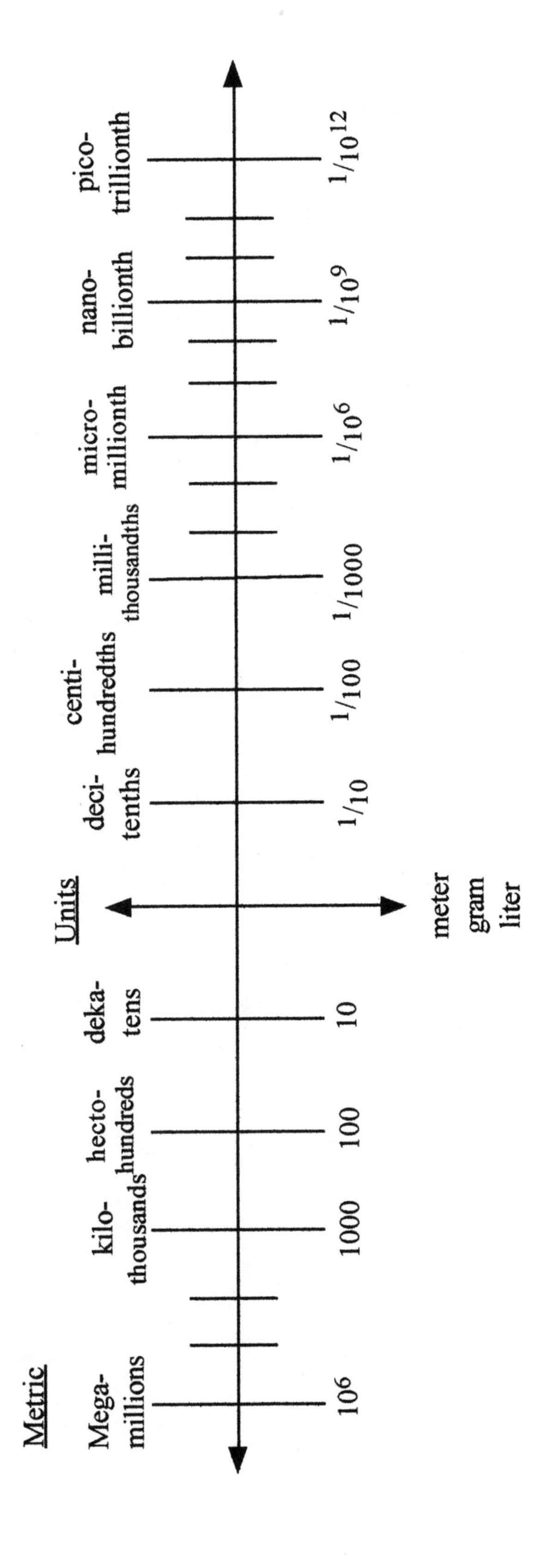
Metric
Mega-
millions
10^6
kilo-
thousands
1000
hecto-
hundreds
100
deka-
tens
10
Units
meter
gram
liter
deci-
tenths
$1/10$
centi-
hundredths
$1/100$
milli-
thousandths
$1/1000$
micro-
millionth
$1/10^6$
nano-
billionth
$1/10^9$
pico-
trillionth
$1/10^{12}$

Practice Set X - 2

Write the abbreviation and the value of the number of units for each of the following:

Metric Units	Abbreviation	Value
(a) kilometer	**km**	**1000 meters**
(b) decimeter	________	________________
(c) milligram	________	________________
(d) dekagram	________	________________
(e) meter	________	________________
(f) deciliter	________	________________
(g) dekameter	________	________________
(h) gram	________	________________
(i) hectometer	________	________________
(j) decigram	________	________________
(k) centiliter	________	________________
(l) liter	________	________________
(m) dekaliter	________	________________
(n) hectoliter	________	________________
(o) kiloliter	________	________________
(p) milliliter	________	________________
(q) centimeter	________	________________

Conversion from one unit to another

As explored briefly in Chapter 8, conversion from one unit to another involves merely moving the decimal point the same number of "steps" in the same direction as it takes to get from one unit to the other.

Examples: (1) 8 km = _?_ cm

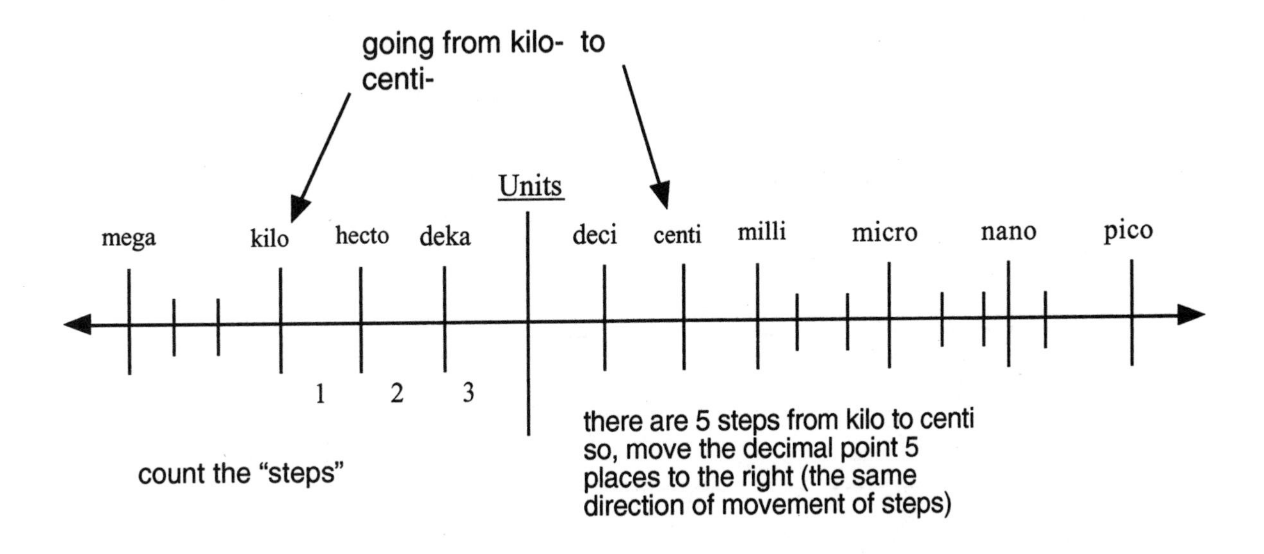

Thus, 8 km = 800000 cm

(2) 4000.2 mg = _?_ kg

That's six steps to the left. Move the decimal point the same 6 places to left.

4000.2 mg = _?_ kg

← move 6 places in this direction

Result? 0.0040002 kg

Practice Set X - 3

Determine the conversion from one unit to another for each of the following:

(a) 0.12 km = ______________________________ dm

(b) 12.0 g = ______________________________ mg

(c) 0.21 hl = ______________________________ cl

(d) 1.5 cm = ______________________________ mm

(e) 5.51 dkg = ______________________________ cg

(f) 0.6125 hg = ______________________________ mg

(g) 3.0 kl = ______________________________ L

(h) 401.0 L = ______________________________ cl

(i) 515.12 dkl = ______________________________ ml

(j) 12.14 km = ______________________________ m

(k) 11.2 mg = ______________________________ dg

(l) 2.1 dl = ______________________________ kl

(m) 12.3 mm = ______________________________ m

(n) 51 g = ______________________________ kg

(o) 23.5 cm = ______________________________ dkm

(p) 65.3 L = ______________________________ hl

(q) 3.4 m = ______________________________ km

(r) 63.5 dm = ______________________________ dkm

(s) 151123.5 ml = ______________________________ kl

Chapter 11

The English and Apothecary Systems

Objectives

Upon completion, the student must be able to do the following:

- **List all abbreviations for each unit.**
- **Make conversions within and between systems.**

Medicines, as well as other materials, are often measured using an antiquated system called the apothecaries' system. It is essential for veterinary medical technologists to be as familiar with this system as with the metric system since each of these systems of measurement will be encountered in the laboratory and in the clinic.

The following are the units and abbreviations of length, volume, and weight. They should be studied and learned.

Length	Volume	Weight
Inches - in.	Fluid Ounces - fl. oz.	Grains - gr.
Feet - ft	Pints - pts	Ounces - oz
Yards - yds	Quarts - qts	Pounds - lbs
Miles - mi	Gallons - gal	Tons - T

There are household measurements with which you should be familiar.

Cups - c   Tablespoons - Tbs or Tbsp or T   Teaspoons - tsp; or t

Length	Weight
12 in = 1 ft	16 oz = 1 lb.
36 in = 1 yd	2000 lb = 1 ton
3 ft = 1 yd	450 gr = 1 oz
5,280 ft = 1 mi	1 oz = 1 fl oz (water)

Volume

16 fl oz = 1 pt	1 pt = 2 cups
32 fl oz = 1 qt	1 qt = 4 cups
2 pt = 1 qt	2 Tbs = 1 fl oz
4 qt = 1 gal	3 tsp = 1 Tbs
8 pt = 1 gal	6 tsp = 1 fl oz
128 fl oz = 1 gal	1 cup = 8 fl oz
	1 pt = 1 lb (liquid)

$$C = \frac{5}{9}(F - 32) \qquad F = \frac{9}{5}C + 32$$

Approximate Equivalents

1 g = 15 gr	1 cup = 240 ml	1 in = 2.5 cm
60 mg = 1 gr	1 fl oz = 30 ml or 30 cc	1 m = 39.4 in
30 g = 1 oz	1 tsp = 5 cc	1 m = 1 yd
454 g = 1 lb	1 pt = 500 ml = 0.5 L	
1 kg = 2.2 lb	1 qt = 1000 ml = 1 L	
	1 gal = 4000 ml = 4 L	
	1 Tbs = 15 ml	

Practice Set XI - 1

Write the abbreviation or the name for each of the following:

1) pint _______ 6) T _______ 11) cup _______

2) lb _______ 7) t _______ 12) mile _______

3) oz _______ 8) fluid ounce _______ 13) ounces _______

4) yard _______ 9) gallon _______ 14) qt _______

5) inch _______ 10) feet _______ 15) grains _______

Sometimes it is necessary to convert from one unit to another. Unlike the metric system, this conversion is often difficult and laborious. Since it is not based on unit of ten, the decimal point cannot be moved to obtain the answer. One must use ratio and proportion or conversion factors to convert units.

Example: Convert 2.5 gal into qt

1 gal = 4 qt

ratio / proportion

$$\frac{xqt}{2.5gal} = \frac{4qt}{1gal}$$

$$xqt = \frac{4qt \times 2.5\cancel{gal}}{1\cancel{gal}}$$

$$x = 10qt$$

conversion

conversion factor: $\frac{4qt}{1gal}$

$$x = 2.5\cancel{gal}\left(\frac{4qt}{1\cancel{gal}}\right)$$

$$x = 10qt$$

Example using multiple conversion factors:

Convert 7 pts to cups.

16 oz (cancelled, 2)	1 cup	7 pts (cancelled)
1 pt (cancelled)	8 oz (cancelled, 1)	

Cancel (top/bottom) units and any numbers that divide evenly (like doing fractions). Your answer will be in the remaining units - Cups. Multiply across the top and bottom and simplify for the quantity.

7 pints is equal to 14 cups

Practice Set XI - 2

Convert the following into the desired units:

a. 2.5 gal = ____________________ qts

b. 256 fl oz =____________________ gal

c. 6 T = ____________________ t

d. 27 fl oz = ____________________ T

e. 5 pts = ____________________ c

f. 2.5 lbs = ____________________ oz

g. $2\frac{1}{4}$ ft = ____________________ in

h $4\frac{1}{3}$ yd = ____________________ ft

i. 18 fl oz = ____________________ tsp

j. 14 ft = ____________________ in

k. 3 oz = ____________________ gr

l. 1.5 qt = ____________________ fl oz

m. 2 mi = ____________________ ft

n. 1.7 tons = ____________________ lbs

o. 3 tablespoons = ______________ tsp

p. 25 oz = ____________________ lbs

Practice Set XI - 3

Convert:

a. 16 fl oz ____________ pts

b. 32 fl oz ____________ pts ____________ qts

c. 128 fl oz ____________ pts ____________ qts ____________ gals

d. 3 gals ____________ qts ____________ pts ____________ fl oz

e. 16 oz ____________ lbs

f. 3 lbs ____________ oz

g. 6 ft ____________ in

h. 36 ft ____________ yds

i. 7 in ____________ ft

j. 72 oz ______________ lbs

k. 3 Tbsp ______________ fl oz

l. 1 Tbsp ______________ tsp

m. 1 tsp ______________ T

n. 30 fl oz ______________ tsp

o. 30 fl oz ______________ tablespoons

p. 8 oz ______________ lbs

q. 24 lbs ______________ oz

r. 10 Tbsp ______________ tsp

Practice Set: XI - 4

Convert:

a. 8 fl oz ______________ pts

b. 2 pts ______________ fl oz

c. 48 fl oz ______________ qts

d. 24 qts ______________ gal

e. 1.5 lb ______________ oz

f. 18 oz ______________ lb

o. 4 pts ______________ qts

p 1.5 pts ______________ fl oz

q. 16 qts ______________ gal

r. 3 pts ______________ gal

s. 0.6 lb ______________ oz

t. 3.5 pts ______________ cups

g. 1 qt ______________ cups

h. 4 fl oz ______________ Tbsp

i. 1 cup ______________ fl oz

j. 1 ton ______________ oz

k. 8 tsp ______________ cups

l. 250 fl oz ___________ gal

m. 5 pts ______________ qts

n. 35 fl oz ___________ qts

u. 1 Tbsp ____________ tsp

v. 4 cups ______________ pts

w. 3 Tbsp ______________ tsp

x. 5 Tbsp ______________ fl oz

y. 2 cups ______________ pts

z. 20 pts ______________ gal

aa. 5 pts ______________ fl oz

bb. 10 fl oz ____________ Tbsp

Chapter 12

The Metric, Apothecary and English Systems

Approximate Equivalents

Objectives

Upon completion, the student must be able to do the following:

- **List the approximate equivalents in common use.**
- **Convert between systems.**

It is often necessary to convert from the metric to the apothecaries' system (or back). For example, if an oral medicine (liquid) is listed in mg per kg or lb; this will have to be converted into the appropriate number of teaspoons or cc's in order for the client to administer the correct prescribed dosage.

The equivalents used are usually only approximations. This provides a generally sufficient accuracy for clinical work. (In a scientific laboratory, for example a research lab, these equivalents as shown here would not be acceptable.) Generally, the accuracy is within 10%.

Example:

Actual	Clinical Usage
1 qt. = 946 ml	1 qt = 1000 ml = 1 L

Example:

It is common to use the following measures for cups/milliliters

1 cup = 240 ml and 1 pt = 500 ml but 1 pt = 2 cups

Of course, there is no substitute for good judgment. One should not convert gallons to milliliters and then the milliliters to fluid ounces (inter-system).

1 gal = 4000 ml = 133 fl oz

It is easier, more efficient, and more accurate to convert directly from gallons to fluid ounces (intra-system).

1 gal = 128 fl oz

Still, there are occasions when you must convert from one value to another, from one system to another, or even make several conversions at a time. However, this should be done only as a last resort or when no better alternative is available.

Q. 1 L = ??? tsp

A. 1 L = 1000 ml = 200 tsp

The conversion from one system to another is generally best performed using ratios and proportions; or by using a conversion factor. Note the similarity to the metric conversions in an earlier chapter.

Example: Convert 2.5 L to gallons

Ratio and Proportion

$$\frac{x}{2.5L} = \frac{1gal}{4L}$$

$$\frac{2.5\cancel{L} \cdot 1gal}{4\cancel{L}} = x$$

x = 0.63 gal

Conversion Factor

$$x = 2.5L\left(\frac{1gal}{4L}\right)$$

x = 0.63 gal

Approximate Equivalents

1 g = 15 gr

60 mg = 1 gr

28.3 g = 1 oz

454 g = 1 lb

1 kg = 2.2 lb

100°C = 212°F (water boils)

37°C = 98.6°F (human body temp)

0°C = 32°F (water freezes)

–17.7°C = 0°F

–40°C = –40°F

1 cup = 240 ml

1 tsp = 5 cc

1 qt = 1000 ml = 1 L

1 Tbsp = 15 ml

1 fl oz = 30 ml or 30 cc

1 pt = 500 ml = 0.5 L

1 gal = 4000 ml = 4 L

1 in = 2.5 cm = 25 mm

1 m = 39.4 in = 3.3 ft

1 m = 1 yd +

1 oz = 480 grains

1 oz = 8 drams

1 dram = 60 grains

1 fl oz = 8 fl drams

1 fl dram = 60 minims (drops)

Example: Convert 75 grains into ounces.

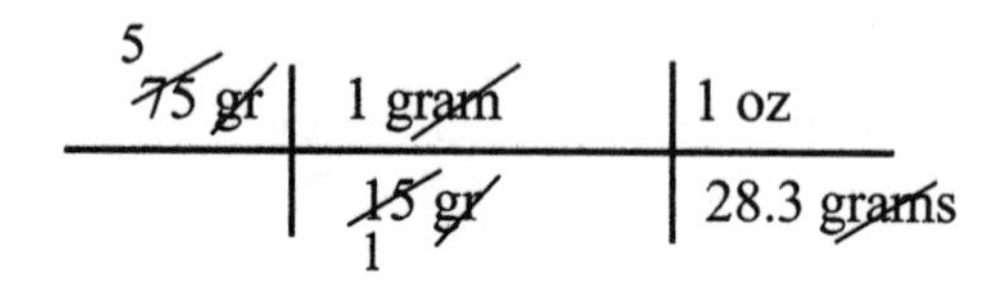

Cancel the units and any numbers. Multiply across the top and across the bottom and simplify.

$5 \div 28.3 = 0.2$ oz

Practice Set XII - 1

Convert:

(a) 35 ml = __________ tsp

(b) 5 in = __________ cm

(c) 2700 ml = __________ qt

(d) 45 g = __________ oz

(e) 3 g = __________ gr

(f) 2 lb = __________ g

(g) 4.5 L = __________ gal

(h) $3\frac{1}{2}$ fl oz = __________ cc

(i) 3 Tbsp = __________ cc

(j) 2.4 gr = __________ mg

(k) 27 kg = __________ lbs

(l) 3 m = __________ in

Temperature Conversion

The two most common temperature scales are *Celsius* and *Fahrenheit.*

To convert from Fahrenheit to Celsius: $C = \frac{5}{9}(F - 32)$

To convert from Celsius to Fahrenheit: $F = \frac{9}{5}C + 32$

The boiling point of water is 212° F or 100° C. Each of these represents the same temperature needed to boil water. Each merely represents a different scale of measurement. The freezing point of water is 32° F or 0° C. Both describe the same condition with regards to heat (or lack of heat = cold.)

To convert from one temperature scale to another, use the given formula, substitute the known value and simplify.

Examples:

F → C

70° F = ? C

$C = \frac{5}{9}(70° - 32°)$

$C \approx 21.1°$

C → F

18° C = ? F

$F = \frac{9}{5}(18°) + 32°$

$F = 64.4°$

Practice Set XII - 2

Convert (round to nearest tenth degree where necessary):

a. 40° C = ___________°F

b. 60° F = ______________°C

c. 37° C = ___________°F

d. 65° F = ______________°C

e. 32° F = ___________°C

f. 70° F = ______________°C

g. 45° F = ___________°C

h. 73° F = ______________°C

i. 100° F = ___________°C

j. 78° F = ______________°C

k. 0° F = ______________°C

l. 80° C = ______________°F

m. -40° C = ___________ °F

n. 100° C = ______________°F

o. -10° F = ____________ °C

p. 80° F = ____________ °C

q. 25° C = ____________ °F

r. 50° C = ____________ °F

s. 10° F = ____________ °C

t. 18° C = ____________ °F

Practice Set XII - 3

Convert as indicated (round to hundredths if necessary):

a. 3 g = ____________ gr

b. 5 oz = ____________ g

c. 130 mg = ____________ gr

d. 4.5 oz = ____________ g

e. 3 oz = ____________ g

f. 35 ml = ____________ **tsp**

g. $2\frac{1}{2}$ lbs = ____________ g

h. 5 lb = ____________ kg

i. 2.5 cups = ___________ cc

j. 8 fl oz = ___________ ml

k. 4 tsp = ___________ ml

l. 3 pts = ___________ ml

m. 7.5 pts = ___________ L

n. 45 ml = ___________ Tbsp

o. 12 in = ___________ cm

p. 350 g = ___________ lbs

q. 45 g = ___________ oz

r. 55 ml = ___________ fl oz

s. 100 ml = ___________ fl oz

t. 3 tsp = ___________ ml

u. 3 Tbsp = ___________ ml

v. 5 pts = ___________ L

w. 85 ml = ___________ tsp

x. 85 ml = ___________ Tbsp

y. 15 ml = ____________ tsp

z. 45 gr = ____________ oz

aa. 100 g = ____________ oz

bb. 300 mg = __________ gr

cc. 13 g = ____________ gr

dd. 220 gr = __________ g

Practice Set XII - 4

Convert:

a. 32 oz = ____________ lbs

b. 18 pts = ____________ qts

c. 16 pts = ____________ gal

d. 6 tsp = ____________ Tbsp

e. 8 tsp = ____________ ml

f. 1 gal = ____________ ml

g. 6 tsp = ____________ Tbsp

h. 3 cups = __________fl oz

i. 3 pts = ____________ cups

j. 12 cups = ____________ pts

k. 45 ml = ____________ Tbsp

l. 1 cup = ____________ fl oz

m. 5 ml = ____________ tsp

n. 3 oz = ____________ g

o. 10 ml = ____________ Tbsp

p. 3 gr = ____________ mg

q. 500 ml = ____________ pts

r. 5 g = ____________ gr

s. 1000 ml = ____________ pts

t. $1\frac{1}{2}$ g = ____________ gr

u. 12 L = ____________ qts

v. 7 ml = ____________ tsp

w. 200 ml = ____________ qts

x. $2\frac{1}{2}$ fl oz = ____________ Tbsp

y. 6 pts = ____________ qts

z. 150 mg = ____________ gr

aa. 13 qts = ____________ gal

bb. 48 g = ____________ oz

cc. 12 ml = ____________ tsp

dd. 85 gr = ____________ g

ee. 12 ml = ____________ Tbsp

ff. 30 ml = ____________ Tbsp

gg. 750 ml = ____________ pts

hh. 45 g = ____________ oz

ii. 5 oz = ____________ g

jj. 6 qts = ____________ fl oz

kk. 2 fl oz = ____________ ml

ll. 5 tsp = ____________ ml

mm. 7 Tbsp = ____________ ml

nn. 1.5 tsp = ____________ ml

Practice Set XII - 5

Convert:

a. 5 cg = ____________ g

b. 1 g = ____________ mg

c. 2 cups = ____________ pints = ____________ qts = ____________ cc

d. 1 pint = ____________ qts

e. 500 cc = ____________ liters

f. 2.5 L = ____________ ml = ____________ cc

g. 0.25 L = ____________ ml

h. 0.1 g = ____________ mg

i. 1 fl oz = ____________ ml

j. 1 qt = ____________ fl oz

k. 1 g = ____________ grains

l. 4 cups = ____________ cc = ____________ pts = ____________ qts

m. 5 cc = ______________ tsp

n. 1 g = ______________ mg

o. 6 fl oz = ______________ cc

p. 2 kg = ______________ lbs

q. 150 mg = ______________ g

r. 1 gr = ______________ mg

s. 1 gal = ______________ qts = ___________ pts = ______________ cc

t. 8 g = ______________ mg

u. 0.5 g = ______________ mg

v. 600 cc = ______________ L

w. 250 mg = ____________ g

x. 1000 mg = ____________ g

y. 15 g = ____________ cg

z. 11 kg = ____________ lbs

aa. 1000 cc = ____________ L

bb. 32 fl oz = ____________ qt

cc. 2 g = ____________ gr

dd. 4000 cc = ____________ gal

ee. 4 pts = ____________ qts

Chapter 13

Word Problems: Dosage and Inter-System Conversion

Objectives

Upon completion, the student must be able to do the following:

- **Read and interpret labels and printed material found in the clinic.**
- **Determine correct dosage.**
- **Accurately calculate and make necessary conversions.**

The technician must be able to locate the desired necessary information, determine the concentration, and calculate the proper dosage. For each of the following problems, use the given information to answer the questions.

Example:

A horse with symptoms of pneumonia is to be treated with a sulfa drug. Determine the proper dose(s) for the 900 pound horse.

Drug	Use	Dosage	Species	Patient
(a) sulfadimethoxine 400 mg/ml	for pneumonia 1 ml/ 16 lb	55 mg/kg	horse	900 lb horse

900 lbs = 409.1 kg

$$\frac{55\ mg}{1\ kg} = \frac{x}{409.1\ kg} \qquad \frac{400\ mg}{1\ ml} = \frac{22500.5\ mg}{x}$$

$$x = 22{,}500.5\ mg \qquad x = 56.25\ ml$$

The horse should receive a dose of 56.25 ml of the drug at the concentration given.

Practice Set XIII - 1

Write a problem using the given information. Solve the problem.

Drug	Use	Dosage	Species	Patient
(a) V-Estravarin Anestrous		0.1 ml/5 lb	dog	35 lb dog
(b) Mannitol 20%	CNS injury	1.5 - 2.0 g / kg 8 ml/kg of 20% sol	dogs & cats	4 kg cat
(c) Electrosulf-3 (1 lb pkg)	pneumonia	(in drinking water) 8 oz/25 gal water Use 1 gal medicated water for each 100 lb B.W. per day for 4 days	calves	150 lb calf

Drug	Use	Dosage	Species	Patient
(d) Erythro-200 (injection: 200 mg/ml)	pneumonia	2 mg/lb daily	swine	500 lb hog
(e) Dextran 6%	plasma expander for shock	up to 200 ml/kg over a period of 24 hours	dogs & cats	55 kg dog
(f) Liquamycin (50 mg/ml)	infections	2 mg/ lb	cattle/horses	1100 lb horse
(g) Hava Span Boluses	pneumonia	1 bolus/ 100 lb for 6 days (dose lasts 48 hours)	cattle	1200 lb cow

Practice Set XIII - 2

Solve the following problems:

(a) Use acepromazine for a preanesthetic:

dosage rate: 0.25 mg / lb
concentration: 10 mg / ml
weight of dog: 50 lbs

(i) dosage in mg: ______________ (ii) dosage in ml: ______________

(b) Induce anesthesia in a 12 lb cat using 4% Surital at a dosage rate of 3 mg / lb

(i) How many mg are needed? ________

(ii) How many ml are needed? ______________

(c) A 20 lb dog with a urinary tract infection will be treated with Gentomycin sulfate at the rate of 2 mg / lb twice a day for 5 days. The concentration of Gentomycin is 50 mg per ml. Determine:

(i) dosage mg each treatment: ______________

(ii) number of ml for each treatment: ________________

(iii) Total number of ml necessary for 5 days: ______________

(d) Tetracycline is dosed at 5 mg per lb every 8 hours. (i) How many 250 mg capsules will a 50 pound dog need daily? _______________ (ii) What are the total number of capsules to be dispensed for 7 days of treatment? ___________________

(e) Calculate the dosage in cc of sodium pentobarbital for each of the following rats if the rate is 5 mg per 100 g and the concentration: 64.8 mg per cc

(i) weight: 250 g (ii) weight: 100 g

(f) Calculate the dosage of sodium pentobarbital for a mouse if the rate is 60 mg / kg and sodium pentobarbital has 64.8 mg per cc. How many cc are needed if the weight of the mouse is

(i) 30 g (ii) 45 g

(g) Calculate the dosage of Vitamin C for a guinea pig. Rate: 2 mg/ 100 g B.W.; Vitamin C has 100 mg / ml. How many ml for each of the given weights of the guinea pigs?

(i) 0.550 kg (ii) 620 g

Practice Set XIII - 3

Given the following information from a label, determine the necessary dosage(s):

(1) **Label**: Whipcide (Phthalofyne)
Each ml contains 250 mg
Sodium bicarbonate sufficient for pH adjustment
Benzyl alcohol 0.01 ml
Water for injection q.s.
Usual dosage: 250 mg (1 ml) per kg

How many cc (dosage) is needed for each of the following dogs:

(i) 45 lb (ii) 15 lb (iii) 22 lb (iv) 83 lb

(2) **Label**: Acepromozine
Each ml contains 10 mg
Usual dosage:
Dogs: 0.25 mg up to 0.5 mg per lb B.W.
Cats: 0.5 mg up to 1.0 mg per lb B.W.
Horses: 2 mg up to 4 mg per 100 lb B.W.

Determine the minimum dosage for each of the following:

(a) Dogs: How many cc for each animal?
(i) 10 kg (ii) 14 kg (iii) 50 kg

(b) Cats: How many cc for each animal?

(i) 1.5 kg (ii) 1 kg (iii) 3.5 kg

(c) Horses: How many cc for each animal?

(i) 500 kg (ii) 350 kg (iii) 900 kg

(3) **Label**: 5 mg/ ml and 2 mg/ kg. How many cc for each of the following dogs:

(i) 24 lbs (ii) 16 lbs (iii) 110 lbs (iv) $5\frac{1}{2}$ lbs

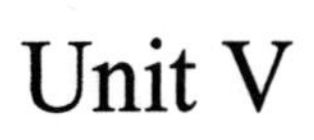
Unit V

Chapter 14

Diluting Solutions and Concentrations

Objectives

Upon completion, the student must be able to do the following:

- **Prepare solutions to any desired concentration.**
- **Dilute solutions as necessary.**

In a laboratory, solutions often are stored in a concentrated form for ease of shipment and storage. The concentrated solution is called the stock solution. The concentration with which the solution is used is often less than this stock concentration. The result is that the technician must be able to dilute, usually with water, these stock solutions to the desired concentration for use. This is accomplished by mixing some certain amount of stock solution with some amount of diluent to achieve the desired concentration.

For example: Isopropyl alcohol (rubbing alcohol) is shipped in concentrations of 100 %. The most effective concentration against bacteria is 70%. (Note that there is an economic factor for buying just one concentration.) The technician must mix the concentrated stock solution (100% alcohol) with water to reach the desired final concentration of 70%.

Note: unless otherwise noted, the diluent is always water.

There are numerous techniques used to determine the correct mix. We present the most widely used and most practical method. Remember that you begin with a concentrated solution and always dilute that solution to the desired concentration. A useful formula is provided:

$$C_1 \cdot V_1 = C_2 \cdot V_2$$

C_1 is the original concentration of the stock solution

V_1 is the volume of the stock solution used

C_2 is the desired (final) concentration (the one you want to make)

V_2 is the volume of the final concentration

Example: You must prepare 4 L of a 70% isopropyl alcohol solution from the 100 % stock solution. You must determine the volume of stock solution to use as well as the diluent, water which must be mixed to achieve 4 liters of total volume.

$$C_1 = 100\% \qquad V_1 = ?$$
$$C_2 = 70\% \qquad V_2 = 4liters$$

determine the known information

$$C_1 \cdot V_1 = C_2 \cdot V_2$$

use the formula

$$100\% \times V_1 = 70\% \times 4liters$$

substitute the known information into the formula

$$V_1 = \frac{70\% \times 4liters}{100\%}$$

cancel the percents; your answer will be in liters

$$V_1 = \frac{280L}{100}$$

$V_1 = 2.8L$ of 100% stock solution of isopropyl alcohol is needed

Now determine the amount of diluent to add (water):

Total volume desired (final volume):	4.0 liters
Amount of (100%) alcohol:	– 2.8 liters
Amount of water needed:	1.2 liters

Example 2: You must prepare as much 40% solution isopropyl alcohol as possible from 2.3 L of 100% stock solution. Determine the volume of 40% solution that can be made and the volume of diluent, water, which is used to make the 40% solution.

$C_1 = 100\%$ $V_1 = 2.3$ L
$C_2 = 40\%$ $V_2 = ???$

Determine the known information

$$C_1V_1 = C_2V_2$$

$$100\% \cdot 2.3\,L = 40\% \cdot V_2$$

$$V_2 = \frac{100\% \cdot 2.3L}{40\%}$$

$$V_2 = 5.75\,Liters$$

Use the formula and substitute the known information. Simplify

Total Volume	5.75 liters
Amount of 100% Alcohol	– 2.3 liters
Amount of water needed	3.45 liters

Practice Set XIV - 1

Solve the following problems and determine the amount of diluent (water, usually) needed

(a) Isopropyl alcohol

	stock	desired	
$C_1 = 100\%$	$V_1 =$ ___???	$C_2 = 70\%$	$V_2 = 2.5$ L

(b) Ethyl alcohol:

$C_1 = 95\%$ $V_1 = \underline{???}$

$C_2 = 70\%$ $V_2 = 3$ L

(c) Formalin (recall that formalin is a liquid):

$C_1 = 10\%$ $V_1 = \underline{???}$

$C_2 = 2\%$ $V_2 = 12$ L

(d) HOAc (acetic acid)

$C_1 = 100\%$ $V_1 = 75$ ml

$C_2 = 2\%$ $V_2 = \underline{???}$

(e) HCl (hydrochloric acid)

$C_1 = 100\%$ $V_1 = 20$ ml

$C_2 = 1\%$ $V_2 = \underline{???}$

(f) $NaHCO_3$ (sodium bicarbonate)

$C_1 = 9\%$ $V_1 = \underline{???}$
$C_2 = 5\%$ $V_2 = 2500$ ml

(g) Isopropyl alcohol

$C_1 = 100\%$ $V_1 = \underline{???}$
$C_2 = 70\%$ $V_2 = 3$ L

(h) EtOH (ethyl alcohol)

$C_1 = 95\%$ $V_1 = \underline{???}$
$C_2 = 70\%$ $V_2 = 5$ l

[recall that liters can be denoted with uppercase L or lowercase l]

(i) NaOH (sodium hydroxide)

$C_1 = 30\%$ $V_1 = 700$ ml
$C_2 = 5\%$ $V_2 = \underline{???}$

(j) Formalin

$C_1 = 100\%$ $V_1 = \underline{???}$
$C_2 = 10\%$ $V_2 = 30\ l$

(k) Formalin

$C_1 = 10\%$ $V_1 = \underline{???}$
$C_2 = 5\%$ $V_2 = 8\ l$

Practice Set XIV - 2

Solve each of the following. Determine the amount of stock solution needed *and* the amount of water to add.

(a) Prepare 30 L of formalin from a 100% stock solution. How much formalin is needed to make:

(i) a 5% solution? (ii) a 1% solution?

(b) A stock solution of NaCl is 9%. Prepare 6 liters of a 0.9% saline solution. How much stock solution is needed?

(c) Ethyl alcohol comes as a 95% stock solution. Prepare:

(i) 6 L of 90%   (ii) 9 l of 70%

(d) Sodium hydroxide has been previously prepared in a concentration of 30% (C_1). But you need a concentration of 5% (C_2) and a volume of 1 L (1000 ml) (V_2). How many ml of the stock solution will you have to use? How much water?

(e) Isopropyl alcohol is 100% but the desired strength is 70%. How much of the 100% stock is needed to make 3 gallons of 70% solution?

(f) If 20 L of alcohol (100%) was available, how many liters of 70% could you make?

(g) 36% HCl needs to be diluted to 1%. Unfortunately there is only 200 ml of HCl left in the lab. How much will this make?

(h) Prepare 25 L of a 10% formalin solution from a 100% stock solution. How much of the stock solution do you need? How much water will you use?

(i) From the 10% formalin solution prepared in (h), make 30 L of: (i) 5% and (ii) 1%. Determine how much stock is needed and the amount of water needed for each.

Practice Set XIV - 3

Solve (You need not compute the amount of diluent):

(1) Isopropyl alcohol

$C_1 = 100\%$	$C_2 = 70\%$
$V_1 = \underline{???}$	$V_2 = 1$ L

(2) EtOH

$C_1 = 95\%$	$C_2 = 70\%$
$V_1 = \underline{???}$	$V_2 = 4$ L

(3) NaOH

$C_1 = 30\%$	$C_2 = 5\%$
$V_1 = 500$ ml	$V_2 = \underline{???}$

(4) Formalin

$C_1 = 100\%$	$C_2 = 10\%$
$V_1 = \underline{???}$	$V_2 = 20$ L

(5) Formalin

$C_1 = 10\%$ $C_2 = 5\%$
$V_1 = \underline{???}$ $V_2 = 5$ L

(6) Formalin

$C_1 = 10\%$ $C_2 = 2\%$
$V_1 = 1$ L $V_2 = \underline{???}$

(7) HOAc

$C_1 = 100\%$ $C_2 = 2\%$
$V_1 = 50$ ml $V_2 = \underline{???}$

(8) HCl

$C_1 = 100\%$ $C_2 = 1\%$
$V_1 = 10$ ml $V_2 = \underline{???}$

Practice Set XIV - 4

$$C_1 \cdot V_1 = C_2 \cdot V_2$$

(1) The isopropyl alcohol on hand is 100%, but the desired strength is 70%. How much of the 100% stock solution is needed to make 2 gallons of 70% solution?

(2) 36% HCl needs to be diluted to 1%. There is 100 ml of HCl on hand. How much will this make?

(3) Make 15 L of a 10% formalin solution from a 100% stock solution. How much of the stock solution is needed? How much water is needed?

(4) From a 10% formalin solution, prepare 20 L of: (i) 5% (ii) 1%

(5) Prepare 20 L of formalin for each of the following from a 100% stock solution,

(i) 5% (ii) 1%

(6) A stock solution of sodium chloride is 9%. From it, prepare 5 L of a 0.9% saline solution.

(7) Ethyl alcohol comes in a 95% stock solution. Prepare:

(i) 5 L of 90% (ii) 7 L of 70%

Chapter 15

Graphs and Graphing Techniques

Objectives

Upon completion, the student must be able to do the following:

- **Understand the basics of graphs and graphing.**
- **Draw and label graphs.**
- **Extract information from a graph.**

A graph is a visual means of presenting numerical data to show relationships between one set of numbers and another. Graphs of data sometimes must be prepared by the technician. Usually the graph will have a vertical axis called the y axis (ordinate) and a horizontal axis called the x axis (abscissa).

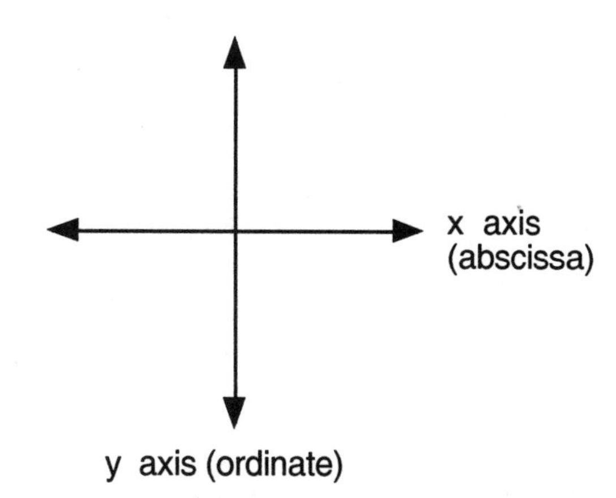

Plotting the graph

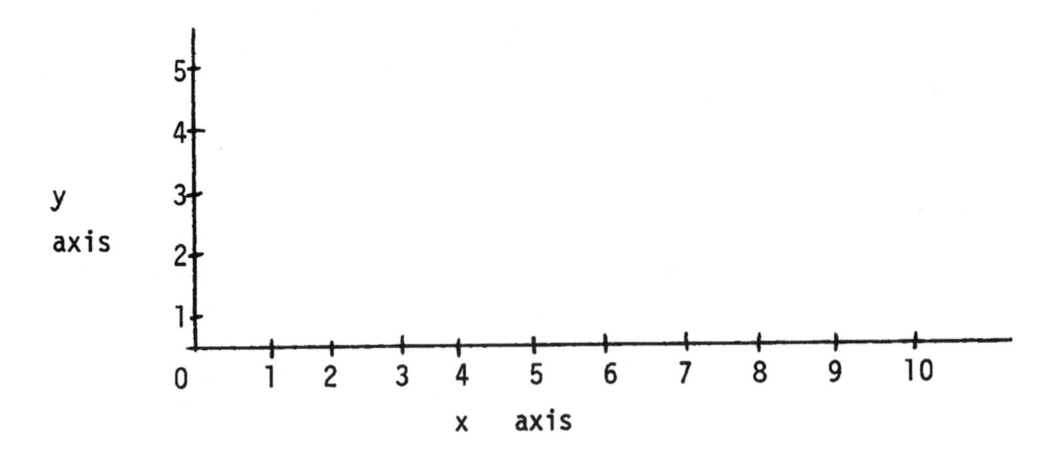

Each axis is divided into the desired units. These units describe some term of the experiment which can be measured. An example might be light absorbed measured on one axis and concentration of a solution measured on the other axis.

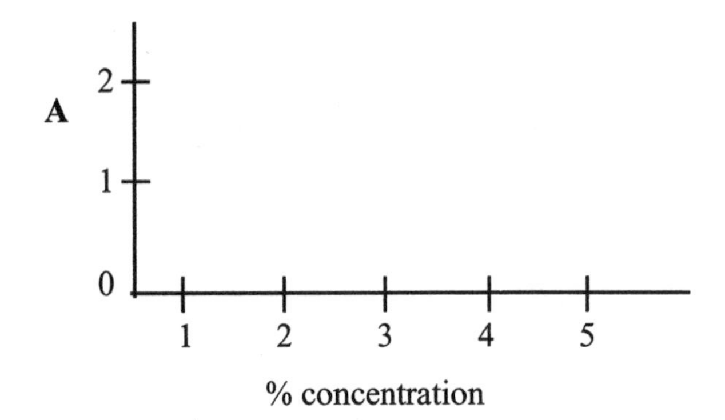

Generally, it makes no difference which is plotted on the x-axis and which is plotted on the y-axis. The divisions are spaced and numbered according to a convenient measurement. In the example shown, (Fig. 15.1) time is measured in minutes and temperature in degrees Celsius. The time scale could have been shown in seconds but the graph would have been larger (much more "spread out"). In this case, the time measurement is on the x-axis and temperature scale is on the y-axis.

Fig. 15.1

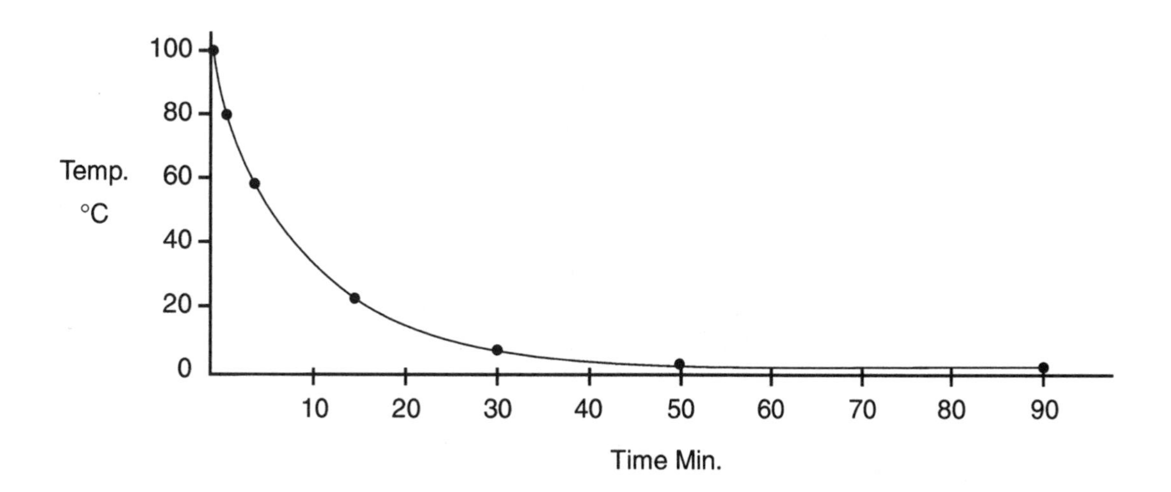

The numbers for the upper limit should be slightly larger than the largest value. You would not select 80 minutes when the last point turned out to be at 90 minutes since this would eliminate some of the data. The lower limit, likewise, must be less than the lowest value. In many cases the lowest value is zero. But be aware of distorted (truncated) graphs which do not start at zero (0). Note, also, that many legitimate graphs do start at some number other than zero.

Some examples of graphs used in Veterinary Medical Technology:

Example 1:

An EKG graph

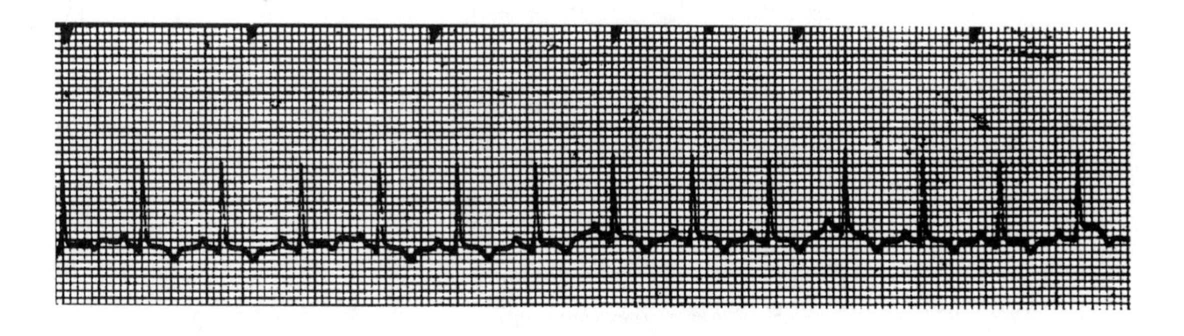

Example 2:

Chart showing respiration rate, heart rate, temperature, and pulse rate.

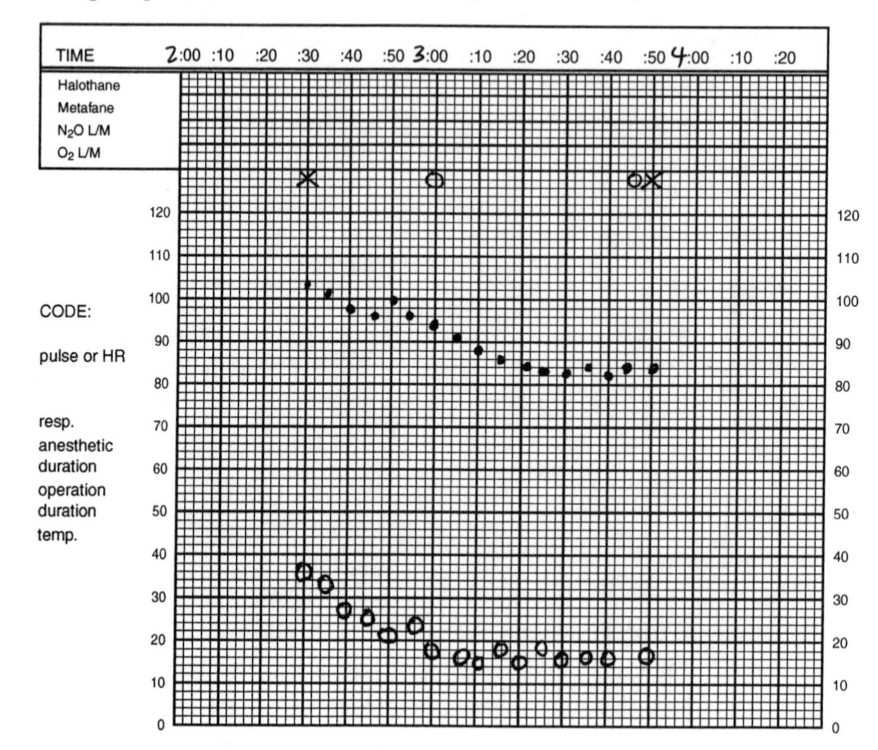

Example 3:

Blood and Urine chemistries are usually line graphs.

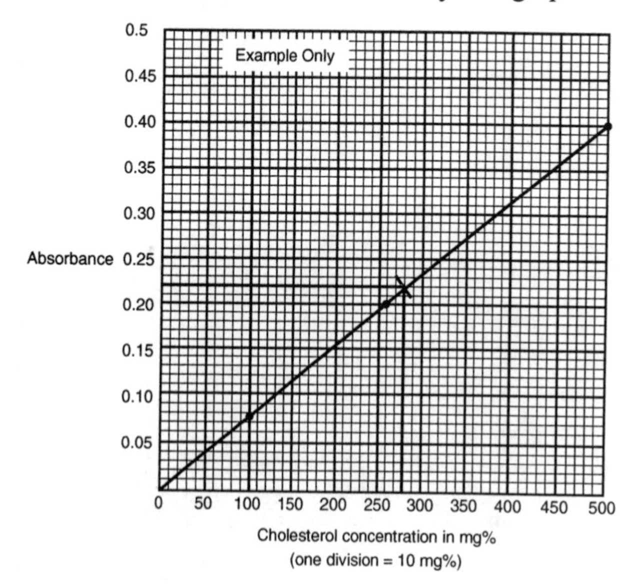

Plotting data on the graph can show changes, trends, and relative quantities.

The x-axis is designated one variable (time, in this example) while the vertical y-axis is designated as another variable (heart rate).

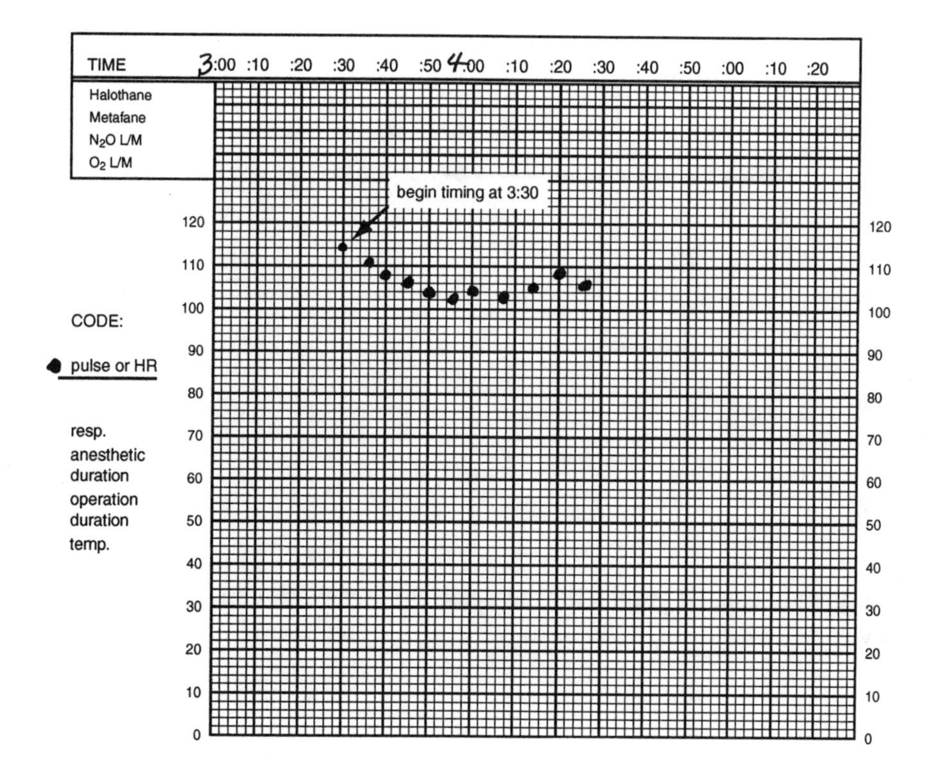

It is common to label each axis with the type of measurement such as time, rate and temperature and also with the respective units (sec, min, beats per min, degrees C).

A two dimensional rectangular graph has four quadrants. The center point is called the origin and is labeled (0, 0). Any point in the plane, that is, on the graph is denoted with an ordered pair of numbers (x, y) which tell the location of that particular point.

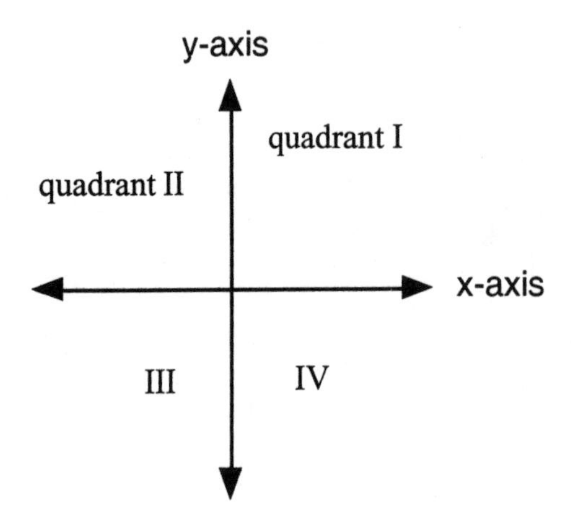

The most common uses of graphs for the veterinary technician involves quadrant I or quadrants I and IV

Examples:

Quadrant I
Blood Chem

A
I
amount

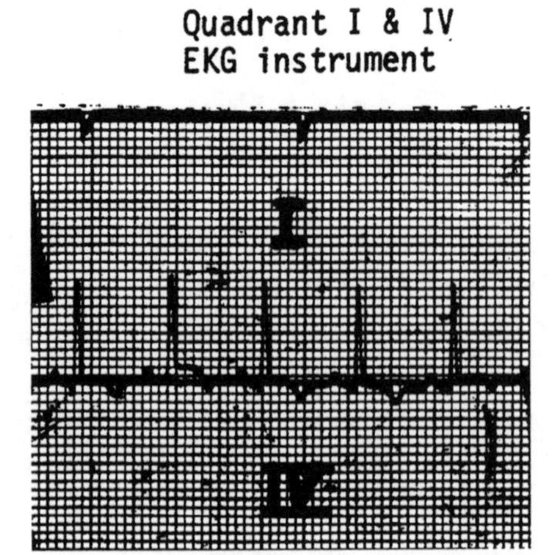

Plotting rectangular coordinates

Plotting in quadrant I. (The most common case.)

All numbers will be positive.

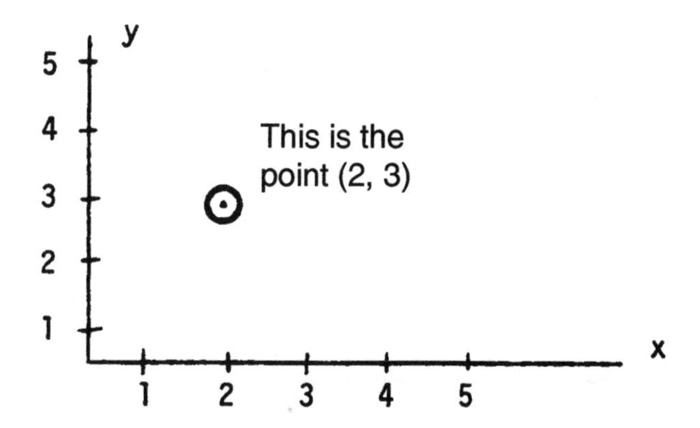

The first value (2) denotes the distance along the x-axis; the second value (3) denotes the distance vertically along the y-axis. The point is plotted where these two meet.

An example best illustrates how to determine where points on graphs should be placed. In this example, use .30 A, which is a measure of the quantity of light absorbed and a concentration of the solution of 3%.

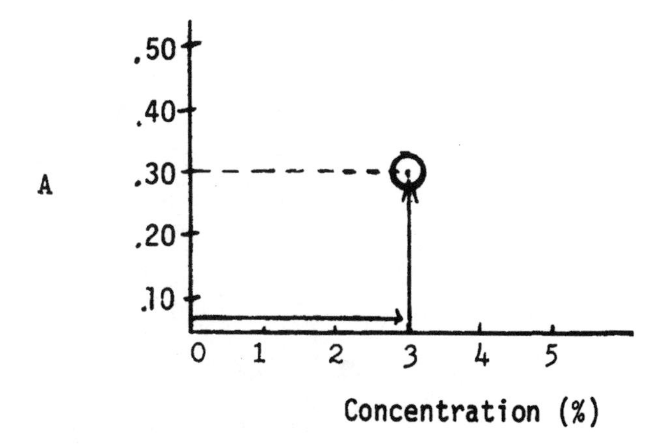

Start at zero (0) and proceeds 3 units to the right along the x-axis. This corresponds to the 3% concentrate. Next, proceed vertically for 3 units which corresponds to .30 on the scale of the y-axis. At this point, make a dot and circle it (as shown.) [It is not absolutely necessary to circle the point like this but is useful at this stage.] The procedure could have been reversed with no effect on the results. Going up 3 units and then over 3 units will yield the same point on the graph.

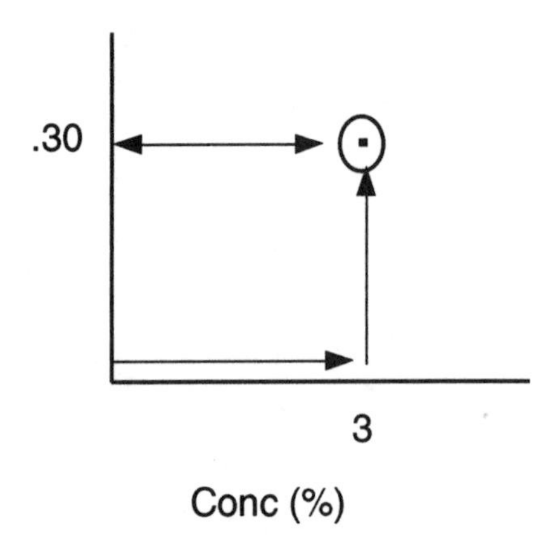

Other known or observed values may be plotted on the same graph. As in the graph example above, the following points are plotted in the same manner. Those points are joined in a straight line.

A	3% Conc
0.1	1
0.2	2
0.3	3
0.4	4
0.5	5

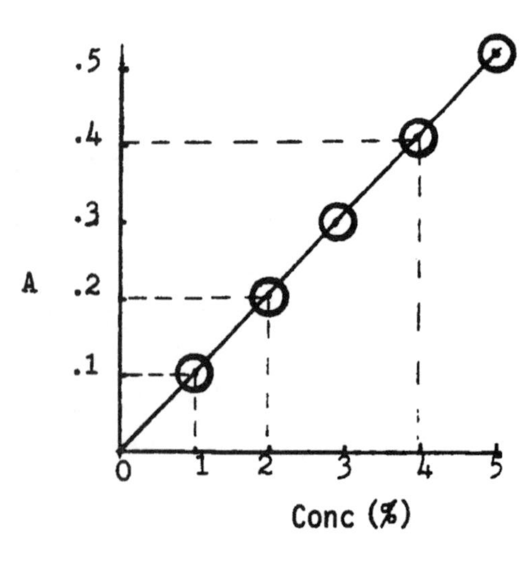

Plotting a Standard Curve (or Standard Plot)

Although referred to as a standard curve it is actually a straight line. It is composed of points derived from known values on both the x- and y-axes.

Several solutions of $CuSO_4$ are made up with known concentrations. The absorbency, A, is then determined using a spectrophotometer. These values are then plotted on a graph.

Example and Practice: Using the given information, plot a standard curve of $CuSO_4$ at wavelength (A).

Concentration vs. A

Conc (%)	A
1	0.05
2	0.10
3	0.15
4	0.20
5	0.25

A

0.3

0.2

0.1

1 2 3 4 5 6 7 8

concentration %

Determining values from an unknown

Once a standard curve has been plotted, it is easy to determine concentrations of other solutions by measuring A using a spectrophotometer. This is the type of determination which is made in the clinical lab.

Example and Practice: Using the standard curve made in the above, the concentration of an unknown $CuSO_4$ is placed in a spectrophotometer and the wavelength, A, is determined. On the graph shown below, (1) go up the y-axis (A) until that value is reached. (2) Then proceed parallel to the x-axis (concentration) until the standard curve is intersected. (3) Now drop vertically to the x-axis to (4) read the corresponding concentration of the solution.

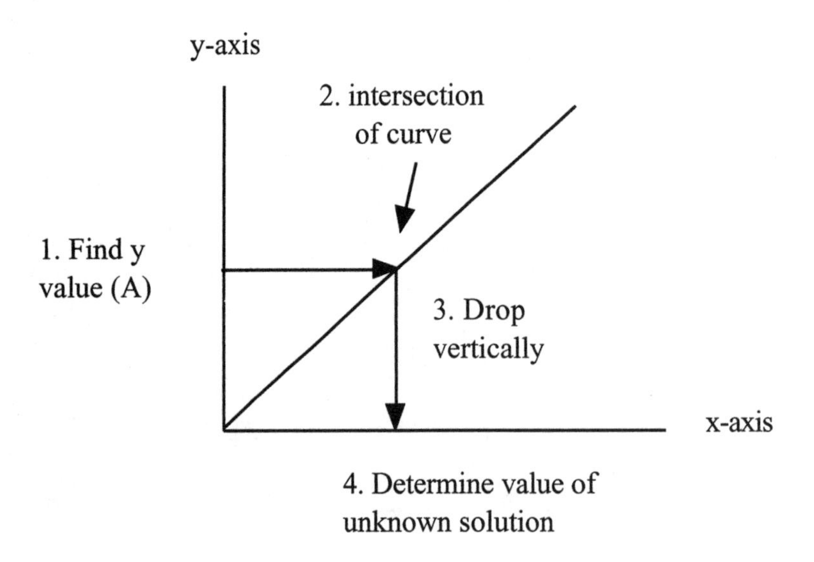

Practice Set XV - I

1. Using the graph of concentration vs. A completed earlier, determine the concentration values for the following solutions.

Information for practice graph

Unknown Solution	A	Concentration
A	0.16	______
B	0.22	______
C	0.15	______
D	0.09	______
E	0.12	______
F	0.24	______

Copy of graph. Include the standard curve you created earlier, then do the exercise above.

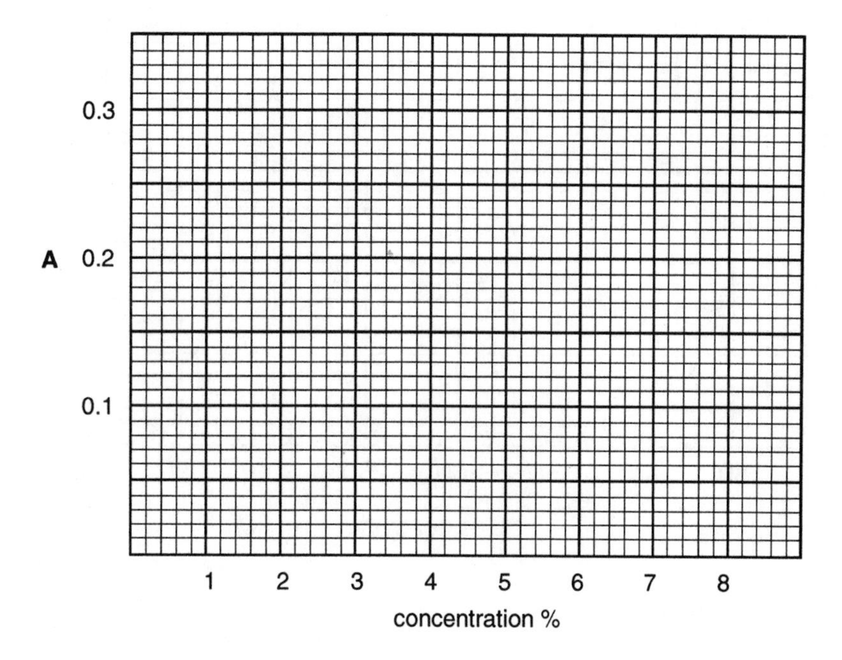

2. Given the following values, plot a standard curve for cholesterol levels.

A	Concentration (mg%)
0.09	100
0.23	260
0.45	500

Absorbency

0.50
0.45
0.40
0.35
0.30
0.25
0.20
0.15
0.10
0.05

0 50 100 150 200 250 300 350 400 450 500

Concentration (mg%)

3. Using the graph constructed on the previous page, determine the concentration of cholesterol in the serum from the graph of the absorbency where (A) are given to be:

Sample	A	mg%
A	0.10	______
B	0.20	______
C	0.30	______
D	0.35	______
E	0.27	______
F	0.18	______

Plotting graphs using quadrants I and IV such as for an EKG

All values along the x-axis are positive. However, y values may be positive or negative. Those y values that lie above the x-axis are positive (in quadrant I) and those below the x-axis are negative (in quadrant IV)

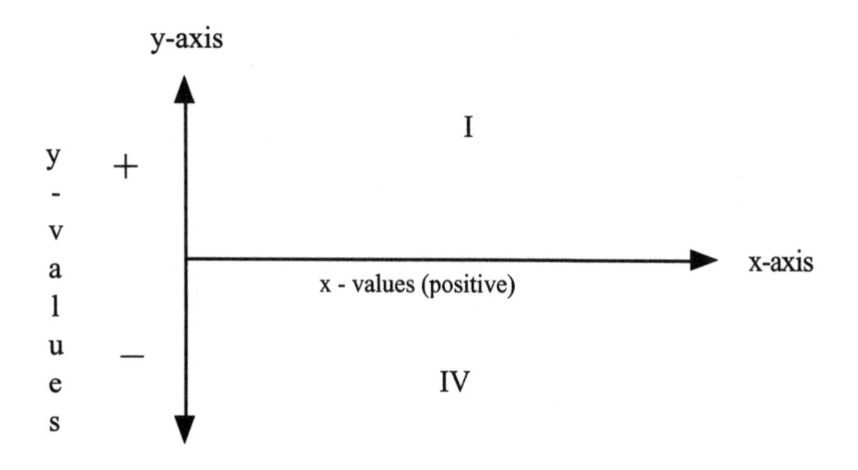

Practice Set XV - 2

1. Recall that coordinates for a point are given as an ordered pair, (x, y). On the graph shown, find the (x. y) values for each lettered point on the graph.

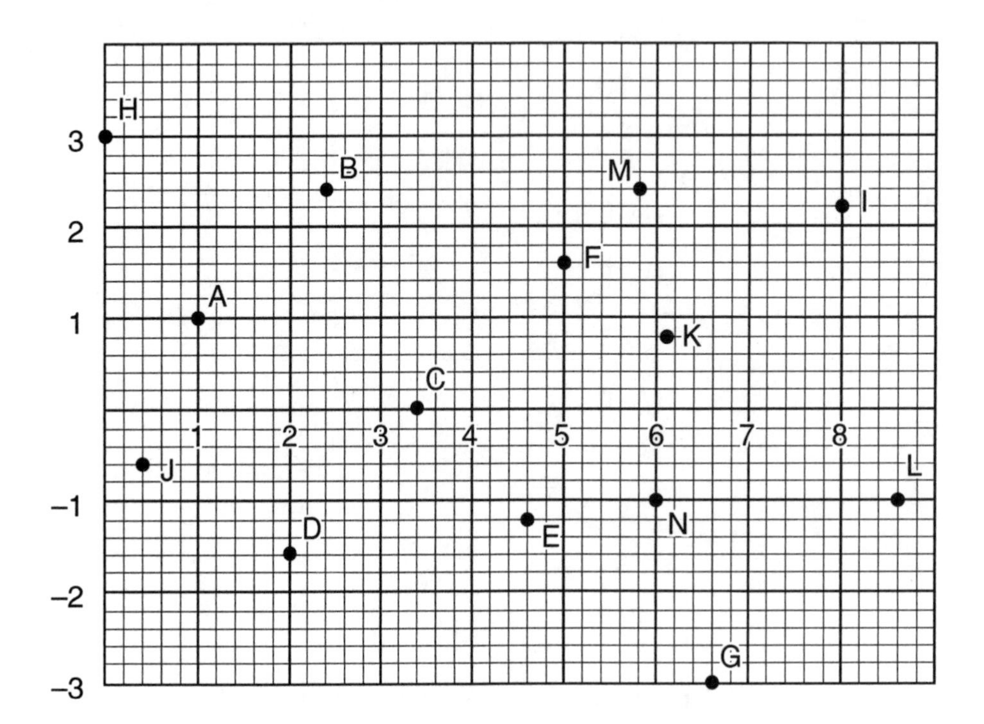

	(x, y)		(x, y)
A	________	H	________
B	________	I	________
C	________	J	________
D	________	K	________
E	________	L	________
F	________	M	________
G	________	N	________

2. The following graph is an example of an EKG recording. Assume 1 cm = 1 MV on the y-axis and 2.5 cm = 1 sec along the x-axis. Determine the millivolt at several positions as indicated by each letter and how much time has elapsed at each letter. The vertical line on the left is 0 seconds.

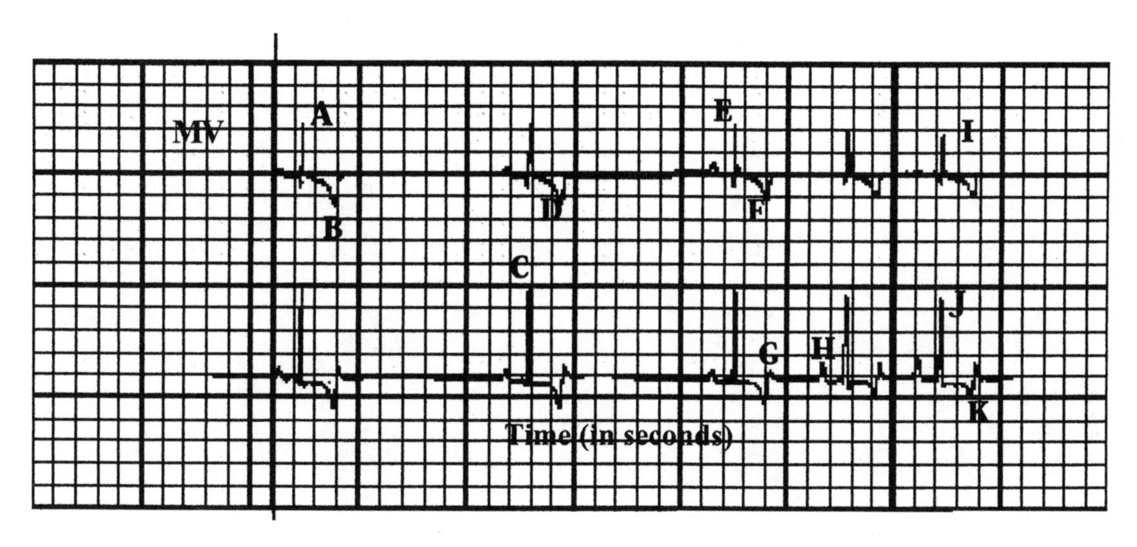

Letter	Time	Millivolt
A		
B		
C		
D		
E		
F		
G		
H		
I		
J		
K		

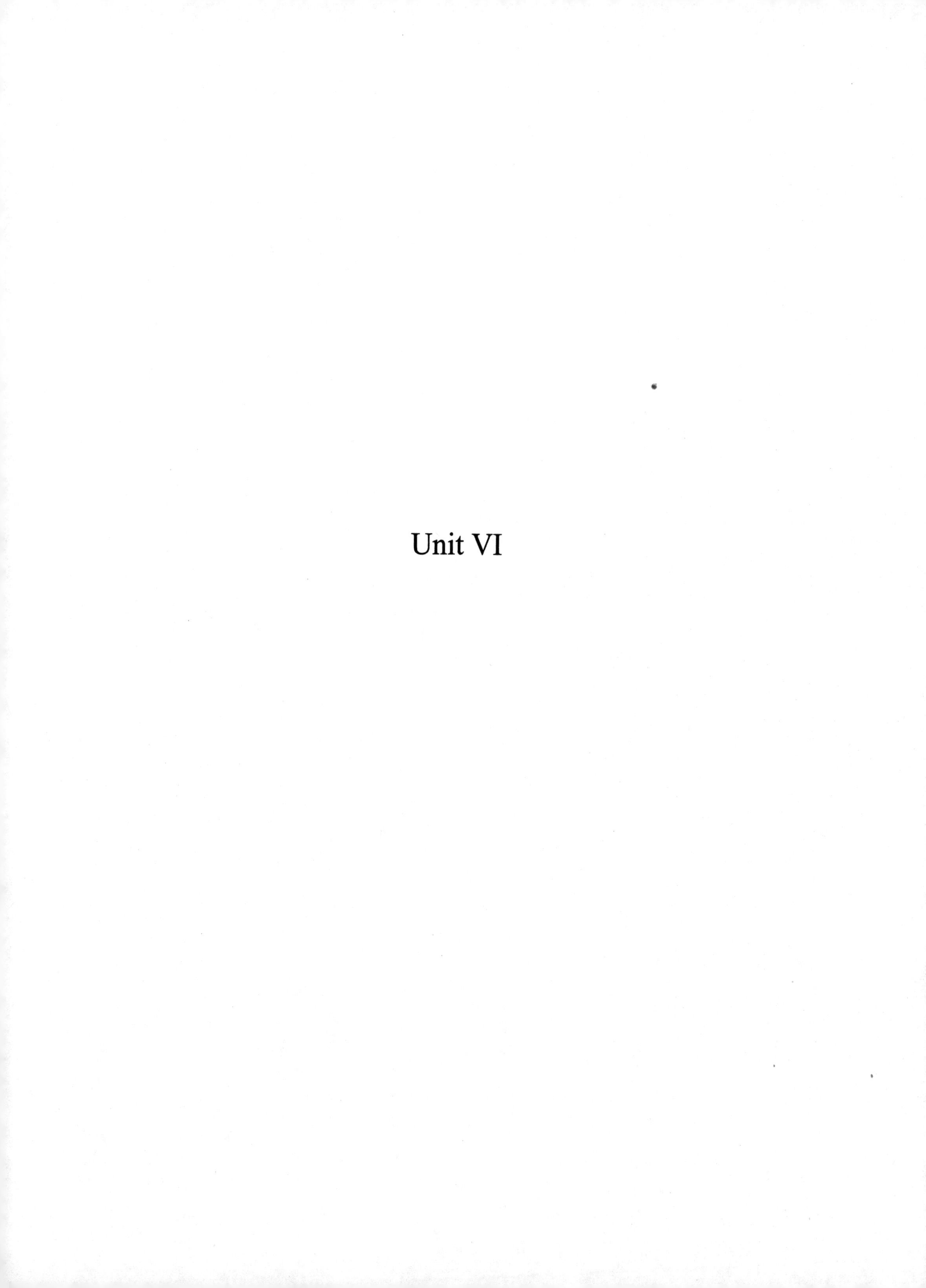

Unit VI

Chapter 16
Statistics

Objectives

Upon completion, the student must be able to do the following:

- **Have a basic understanding of statistics and statistical methods.**
- **Be able to compute simple standard statistical measures.**

In every technical occupation, an understanding of statistics is essential. In this chapter, we explore some of the common statistical concepts, terms, numerical methods, and techniques that will form a basis for understanding. This is meant as an overview and in no way can this one chapter alone provide the technician with the skills they will surely need in a laboratory or clinical setting. A semester course in basic statistics is strongly recommended.

Knowledge of statistics allows you to make educated, informed decisions based upon data (information). Statistics is the study of collecting, organizing, and interpreting numerical information and making decisions based upon that information.

You are probably familiar with some concepts - the average, for example. But what constitutes an average? Here's an example: suppose you were looking at houses and the real estate agent told you the average price of a home for your area was more than $175,000. What does this mean, exactly? Which "average" is the agent referring to?

In statistics there are three common "averages". The *mean*, which is the "average" most people think of when they think of the term average. The mean is arrived at by adding all the relevant items and dividing by how many of those items there are. If you took five tests in this class and scored an 85, 90, 92, 95, and 94 you could compute your mean score. Do that now.

Another type of average is called the *median.* Often, this number is more meaningful than the mean. The median is the middle number of a set of data. When the data is ordered, there are as many numbers above the median as below it. This can be especially important if one or more of the numbers involved is extreme in some way. Suppose on those five tests, you scored a 58 rather than the 90. Again compute your average. In addition, order the numbers, locate the middle number - that is the median. Which of these numbers seems more meaningful? Perhaps you weren't fully prepared for that test on which you got a 58. Or maybe you were ill that day. In any event, that one test had the effect of pulling your average (the mean) down. Yet the median tells a different story. In this case, the median, the middle number, is much more representative of the type of work of which you are capable.

A third type of average is called the *mode*. The mode is the number that occurs most often in a set of data. In the test scores given previously, there was no number that occurred more than any other; thus, no mode.

Example:

Seven houses were sold last week in your area. The houses sold for the following prices: $120, 000; $124, 000; $122, 500; $124, 000; $498,500; $124,000; and $123, 800.

The "average" selling price (rounded to nearest dollar) : $176,686 This is the mean.

($120, 000 + $124, 000 + $122, 500 + $124, 000 + $498,500 + $124,000 + $123, 800) ÷ 7

Or, the "average" selling price : $124, 000 This is the median.

$120,000 $122,500 $123,800 $124,000 $124,000 $124,000 $498,500

middle number

Or, the "average" selling price: $124, 000 This is the mode.

$124, 000 occurs three times

Which of these is representative of the selling prices given?

These averages, called *measures of central tendency* describe how data is grouped. They describe the grouping of data about some central point or measure.

Measures of variation, on the other hand, describe how data is spread out. The *range* is a measure of the difference between the highest data value and the lowest. The measures of *variation* and *standard deviation* tell how much data varies around some middle value.

These measures of variation can describe if the data is all closely grouped or spread widely apart. Standard deviation is the square root of the variance. Many modern calculators perform these statistical functions making it easy to grasp the importance of the data rather than distracting you with tedious computations.

Graphs and charts are another significant aspect of statistics. They have the advantage of presenting data clearly and allowing insight into trends. *Stem-and-leaf plots* are useful for providing a quick "snapshot" of the data as well as preserving all the original data itself. *Histograms* and *scatter plots* provide insights into the relationships among data. Bar graphs, circle graphs and pictograms all provide a useful visual pictures of the data; while several types of line graphs can be used to indicate trends over time. All are useful tools in analyzing information.

A *variable* may take on different values; a single characteristic or trait for example, height, weight, age, blood type, number of telephones in one's home or number of pets one owns. These are all examples of variables. A *random variable* is a variable whose values are due to chance.

Statisticians collect and analyze these variables and look for patterns. Each observation is a data value. The collection of these observations is the data set. Data are the actual observations of the phenomena of interest based upon samples.

A *sample* is some part of the population we can observe. Observation of the sample leads to information on a phenomena of interest. The *population* is the entire universe of possibilities; *all* of the items.

One of the most common errors in statistics involves making specific predictions. We may make a generalization, but we cannot predict specifics. Some reasons for this include:

1. Data set may be too small a sample.
2. Other variables may be present for which you are unaware or had not considered.
3. Problems with observation (for example, people tend to lie on surveys!)

All fields have their own language and notation. Statistics is no different. Some notation typically found in the study of statistics include:

$\bar{x}$ read as x-bar; symbolizes the mean

$\tilde{x}$ read as x-tilde; symbolizes the median

s^2 symbolizes the variance of a sample

s standard deviation; $s = \sqrt{s^2}$ means standard deviation = $\sqrt{\text{variance}}$

Σ sigma (uppercase); summation

Summation notation is used in many statistical formulas. It is a notational device indicating addition and tells the user what should be added and the conditions for the addition.

$$\sum_{i=1}^{n} x_i$$

These are called index numbers; the lower tells where to begin (in this case with the first data value) and the upper tells where to stop (the nth value)

This part tells what is being added and what to do with it; do this part first, then add all the resultant values

In statistics, the index numbers are usually omitted since *all* the data values are used.

Examples:

(1) Given the data: {1, 2, 3, 4, 5, 6}; Determine Σx

This notation tells us to take each value of x, the data set, and then add or sum the result.

$$\Sigma x = 1+2+3+4+5+6 = 21$$

(2) Given {1, 2, 3, 4, 5, 6}; Determine Σx^2

$$\Sigma x^2 = 1^2 + 2^2 + 3^2 + 4^2 + 5^2 + 6^2 = 91$$

Note: in this case, first square each value, then add.

(3) Given {1, 2, 3, 4, 5, 6}; Determine $(\Sigma x)^2$

$$(\Sigma x)^2 = (1+2+3+4+5+6)^2 = (21)^2 = 441$$

Note the difference. In this case, the notation tells us to add the values **first**, then square the result.

Pay particular attention to the distinction between the second and third examples!

Practice Set XVI - 1

1. Given the set of numbers = {4, 8, 9, 2, 5} , Compute:

(a) Σx

(b) $\frac{\Sigma x}{n}$

(c) Σx^2

(d) $\Sigma(x-5.6)$

(e) $\Sigma(x-5.6)^2$

2. Given $x_1 = 12, x_2 = 11, x_3 = 14, x_4 = 13$, Compute:

(a) Σx

(b) Σx^2

(c) $\Sigma(x-1)^2$

Now that you have had a little practice with using summation notation, we are going to introduce some formulas to use in computing statistics. We'll begin with a set of data, say test scores, and explore several important statistical concepts along the way.

Given the following test scores:

66	79	53	65	89	76	73	84	76	69	77	97
75	78	80	71	86	68	64	76	86	72	76	68

Construct a stem-and-leaf diagram. Such a diagram has *stems* on the left of the vertical bar and *leaves* on the right. Since the data are all two-digits, the stems are the tens place while the units will be the leaves.

5	3
6	4 5 6 8 8 9
7	1 2 3 5 6 6 6 6 7 8 9
8	0 4 6 6 9
9	7

A stem-and-leaf diagram has the advantages of being easy to complete and all the original data is preserved. On the other hand, it is not very useful for very large data sets.

The next step is to order the scores from least to greatest. This is a common first step. With the information thus ordered, we can began to make better sense of the data, look for patterns, and perform statistical calculations.

From this we can find the *median*, which is the middle score. The median divides the data into two halves. In some cases, we might want to further divide the data. *Quartiles* divide the data into four equal parts. Closely related to quartiles are percentiles.

Percentiles give an indication of any one individual's score placement as measured against the whole set. The percentile rank indicates how many scored below that rank. That is, if your score was in the 35th percentile that means that 35% of the other people scored below you.

The median corresponds to the 50th percentile as well as the second quartile. The first and third quartiles correspond to the 25th and 75th percentiles, respectively.

Exercise:

Determine the mean, median and the mode for the given scores. Also, find the range, variance and the standard deviation. In the following pages you will find tables of the data values which can be used to determine these measures of central tendency and variation.

Simple formulas for these sample measures include:

$$\textbf{\textit{Mean}} = \frac{\sum x}{n}$$

Variance: $$s^2 = \frac{n\sum x^2 - \left(\sum x\right)^2}{n(n-1)}$$ (Use this computational formula)

The number of data values is __________ ? This value is n.

Ordered scores:

53

64

65

66

68

68

69

71

72

73

75

76

76

76

76

77

78

79

80

84

86

86

89

97

With statistical problems, it is often helpful to organize the data in tables or columns. Since we need to know the sum of all the "X's" and the sum of all the X's squared …

x	x^2	
53	2809	
64	4096	
65	4225	
66	4356	
68	4624	
68	4624	
69	4761	
71	5041	
72	5184	
73	5329	
75	5625	
76	5776	
76	5776	
76	5776	
76	5776	
77	5929	
78	6084	
79	6241	
80	6400	
84	7056	
86	7396	
86	7396	
89	7921	
97	9409	
1804	137610	*Totals*

We are trying to determine the mean, median and mode. The formula for mean is given previously. The mode is the number ______________________________. The median is the ____________________ number and its location (once the values are ordered) can be determined using $\frac{n+1}{2}$. Note that this does *not* give the value for the median, only its location in the ordered numbers. In this case, since n = 24, the median must be between the 12th and 13th numbers. Use the average of these two numbers to locate the median.

The range is the ____________________ between the highest and lowest values. Use the given formula to determine the variance. To find the standard deviation, take the square root of the variance.

Measures of central tendency:

Mean: ___________ Median: ______________ Mode: ________

Measures of variation:

Range:

Variance (use the given formula and the previous tables):

Standard Deviation (take the square root of the number found for the variance):

Practice Set XVI - 2

Circle the correct response: T - True F - False

(a) For the data set: 5, 9, 12, 11, 2, 4, 9, and 8, the range would be 10. T F

(b) A single extremely large value (an outlier) can affect the median more than the mean. T F

(c) Quartiles divide data into four equal groups. T F

(d) If a person's score on an exam corresponds to the 75th percentile, then that person obtained 75 correct answers out of 100 questions. T F

(e) For the sample: 1, 8, 7, 2, 9, 15, and 18, the mean is 7.6. T F

(f) For the sample: 19, 21, 19, 17, 18, 19, and 21, the mode is 19. T F

(g) For the sample: 1.3, 2.7, 8.9, 7.3, 9.2, and 8.1, the median is 8.9. T F

(h) If the values of the data set are near the mean, the variance will be small. T F

(i) If the standard deviation of a distribution is 2.53, the variance is 1.59. T F

(j) The mode is the value that occurs most frequently in a data set. T F

(k) The mean is the value that corresponds to the 50th percentile. T F

Multiple Choice: Circle the letter of the correct response

(l) The notation $\sum_{i=1}^{4} x_i$ means:

(a) 1 X 2 X 3 X 4 (b) 1 + 2 + 3 + 4

(c) x + x + x + x (d) None of the above

(m) Measures of central tendency are quantities which:

(a) numerically describe data. (b) describe the distribution of data.

(c) describe the grouping of data. (d) describe qualitative data.

(n) Measures that describe how the data is distributed or spread out are:

(a) range. (b) variance.

(c) standard deviation. (d) all of the above.

(o) Calculate the range and standard deviation (listed in that order) of the following sample test grades:

87 75 68 57 69 78

(a) 30, 9.3 (b) 30, 10.19 (c) 25, 9.3 (d) 25, 10.19

(p) Variance is a measure that:

(a) shows how the data fluctuates about the median.

(b) shows how the data fluctuates about the mean.

(c) shows how the data fluctuates within the interquartile range.

(d) shows how the data fluctuates within the range.

Practice Set XVI - 3

Solve the following:

(1) Petroleum pollution in oceans is known to increase the growth of a certain bacteria. Sarah did a project for her ecology class in which she made bacteria counts (per 100 milliliters) in nine random samples of sea water. Her counts gave the following readings:

17 23 18 19 21 16 12 15 18

(a) Find the range. ______________

(b) Find the sample mean. ___________

(c) Find the sample standard deviation. ___________

(2) Kennel occupancy rates often dictate how easy it might be to reserve a space at the last minute and determine the average cost of that space. Kennel spaces are often discounted in areas with low occupancy. Occupancy rates across the United States for major cities are given below.

56	89	79	71	70	60	60	61	62	63	64	65
81	73	68	72	56	59	60	62	73	64	72	67

(a) Determine the mean, median and mode

(b) Find the standard deviation

(c) Make a stem-and-leaf plot

Answer Keys

Practice Set I -1

(1) 20
(2) XV
(3) XXX
(4) 26
(5) IX
(6) 23
(7) XXIX
(8) 19
(9) VIII
(10) XVI
(11) 1,179
(12) MCMLXXIII
(13) 64
(14) 99
(15) MCMLXXV
(16) 448
(17) CXII
(18) XLIX
(19) 3,333
(20) MMCCXXII

Practice Set II - 1

(1)
(a) $\frac{2}{4} = \frac{1}{2}$
(b) $\frac{3}{8}$
(c) $\frac{5}{9}$
(d) $\frac{5}{12}$

(2)
(a) $\frac{1}{12}$
(b) $\frac{5}{12}$
(c) $\frac{11}{12}$
(d) $\frac{7}{12}$

(3)
(a) $\frac{1}{36}$
(b) $\frac{35}{36}$
(c) $\frac{13}{36}$
(d) $\frac{19}{36}$

(4)
(a) $\frac{7}{60}$
(b) $\frac{13}{60}$
(c) $\frac{30}{60} = \frac{1}{2}$
(d) $\frac{45}{60} = \frac{3}{4}$

(5)
(a) $\frac{12}{100} = \frac{3}{25}$
(b) $\frac{37}{100}$
(c) $\frac{50}{100} = \frac{1}{2}$
(d) $\frac{99}{100}$

Practice Set II - 2

(a) $\frac{3}{5}$
(b) $\frac{1}{2}$
(c) $\frac{1}{2}$
(d) $\frac{3}{4}$
(e) 4
(f) $\frac{1}{3}$
(g) $\frac{1}{2}$
(h) $\frac{7}{8}$
(i) $\frac{8}{9}$
(j) $\frac{2}{3}$
(k) $\frac{5}{9}$
(l) $\frac{2}{7}$

Practice Set II - 3

1) $3\frac{1}{3}$
2) $3\frac{2}{5}$
3) $6\frac{1}{4}$
4) $4\frac{1}{8}$
5) $2\frac{3}{16}$
6) 4
7) $\frac{13}{3}$
8) $\frac{33}{2}$
9) $\frac{19}{10}$
10) $\frac{37}{7}$
11) $\frac{35}{9}$
12) $\frac{51}{4}$

Practice Set II - 4

1) a) $\frac{1}{4}$ b) $\frac{1}{6}$ c) $\frac{24}{25}$ d) $\frac{1}{4}$ e) $\frac{1}{2}$ f) $\frac{1}{6}$ g) $\frac{1}{8}$ h) $\frac{1}{9}$

2) a) $\frac{71}{8}$ b) $\frac{49}{18}$ c) $\frac{47}{6}$ d) $\frac{29}{8}$ e) $\frac{59}{12}$ f) $\frac{54}{7}$ g) $\frac{62}{9}$ h) $\frac{21}{8}$

3) a) 3 b) $6\frac{6}{7}$ c) $6\frac{1}{9}$ d) $7\frac{1}{9}$ e) $21\frac{1}{4}$ f) $3\frac{4}{7}$ g) $4\frac{1}{5}$ h) $5\frac{1}{4}$

Practice Set III - 1

(a) $1\frac{1}{3}$ (b) $1\frac{1}{4}$ (c) $3\frac{1}{2}$ (d) 4 (e) $2\frac{6}{7}$ (f) $2\frac{1}{2}$ (g) $1\frac{2}{3}$ (h) $8\frac{1}{3}$

Practice Set III - 2

(a) $\frac{1}{9}$ (b) $\frac{1}{16}$ (c) $\frac{1}{12}$ (d) $\frac{4}{27}$ (e) $\frac{3}{10}$ (f) $\frac{6}{25}$ (g) $\frac{15}{32}$ (h) $\frac{21}{40}$

Practice Set III - 3

(a) $\frac{4}{15}$ (b) $\frac{3}{25}$ (c) $\frac{3}{20}$ (d) $\frac{6}{25}$ (e) $\frac{3}{5}$ (f) $\frac{2}{15}$

(g) $\frac{1}{4}$ (h) $\frac{1}{9}$ (i) $\frac{1}{6}$ (j) $\frac{1}{4}$ (k) $\frac{2}{5}$ (l) $\frac{1}{2}$

Practice Set III - 4

(a) $\frac{5}{2}$ (b) $\frac{11}{3}$ (c) $\frac{21}{5}$ (d) $\frac{17}{8}$ (e) $\frac{53}{16}$

Practice Set III - 5

(a) 32 (b) 5 (c) 22 (d) $11\frac{1}{2}$ (e) $13\frac{1}{5}$ (f) $4\frac{1}{5}$ (g) $9\frac{1}{3}$

(h) $10\frac{20}{21}$ (i) $9\frac{4}{5}$ (j) $11\frac{1}{2}$ (k) $56\frac{1}{4}$ (l) $12\frac{11}{12}$ (m) $8\frac{5}{16}$ (n) $14\frac{1}{12}$

Practice Set III - 6

(a) $41\frac{1}{4}$ lbs (b) $280\frac{1}{2}$ lbs (c) 21 lbs (d) $17\frac{5}{8}$ oz

Practice Set III - 7

(a) $\frac{1}{3}$ (b) $\frac{1}{10}$ (c) $\frac{5}{3}$ (d) $\frac{8}{5}$

Practice Set III - 8

(1) 15 (2) 16 (3) 16 (4) 35 (5) 24 (6) 50 (7) 64 (8) 100 (9) 70

Practice Set III - 9

(a) $\frac{5}{6}$ (b) 2 (c) $1\frac{1}{5}$ (d) $\frac{8}{27}$ (e) $\frac{5}{9}$ (f) $1\frac{1}{2}$ (g) $2\frac{1}{10}$ (h) $\frac{2}{3}$ (i) 48 shakers

Practice Set III - 10

(a) $26\frac{2}{3}$ (b) $\frac{4}{5}$ (c) $\frac{13}{30}$ (d) $\frac{2}{3}$ (e) $\frac{1}{4}$ (f) $2\frac{2}{5}$ (g) 18 (h) 5 (i) $1\frac{1}{5}$ (j) 20

Practice Set III - 11

(a) $\frac{7}{9}$ (b) $\frac{1}{2}$ (c) $\frac{2}{5}$ (d) $4\frac{3}{8}$ (e) $\frac{1}{2}$ (f) $7\frac{7}{8}$ (g) $\frac{1}{6}$ (h) 1 (i) $1\frac{1}{2}$ (j) 2

(k) $1\frac{1}{2}$ (l) $1\frac{1}{3}$ (m) $5\frac{1}{3}$ (n) $1\frac{1}{6}$ (o) 12 (p) $4\frac{2}{3}$ (q) 8 (r) $3\frac{16}{25}$ (s) 16 (t) 4

(u) 24 (v) 4 (w) $\frac{1}{4}$ (x) $\frac{152}{275}$ (y) $\frac{10}{29}$ (z) 27 (aa) 8 (bb) 2 (cc) $\frac{8}{25}$ (dd) 1

(ee) 6 (ff) 1 (gg) 1

Practice Set IV - 1

(a) $\frac{7}{8}$ (b) $\frac{10}{16}=\frac{5}{8}$ (c) $\frac{4}{5}$ (d) $\frac{12}{16}=\frac{3}{4}$ (e) $\frac{3}{7}$ (f) $\frac{9}{8}=1\frac{1}{8}$ (g) $\frac{20}{16}=1\frac{4}{16}=1\frac{1}{4}$

Practice Set IV - 2

(a) $\frac{1}{3}$ (b) $\frac{1}{2}$ (c) $\frac{2}{3}$ (d) $\frac{3}{4}$ (e) $\frac{5}{12}$ (f) $\frac{5}{8}$ (g) $\frac{5}{8}$ (h) $\frac{5}{6}$

(i) $\frac{3}{8}$ (j) $\frac{5}{6}$ (k) $\frac{9}{14}$ (l) $1\frac{1}{8}$ (m) $\frac{1}{3}$ (n) $\frac{53}{24}=2\frac{5}{24}$ (o) $\frac{13}{8}=1\frac{5}{8}$ (p) $\frac{257}{120}=2\frac{17}{120}$

Practice Set IV - 3

(a) $13\frac{5}{12}$ (b) $10\frac{7}{10}$ (c) $19\frac{5}{8}$ (d) $17\frac{7}{10}$ (e) $15\frac{3}{4}$ (f) $20\frac{1}{2}$ (g) $22\frac{3}{5}$ (h) $17\frac{5}{8}$

(i) $13\frac{1}{2}$ (j) $19\frac{1}{3}$ (k) $15\frac{1}{2}$ (l) $12\frac{1}{3}$ (m) $16\frac{1}{2}$ (n) $16\frac{7}{8}$ (o) $8\frac{7}{9}$

Practice Set IV - 4

(a) $3\frac{11}{16}$ (b) $4\frac{1}{8}$ (c) $4\frac{17}{20}$ (d) $7\frac{1}{2}$

Practice Set IV - 5

(a) $3\frac{11}{12}$ (b) $12\frac{1}{8}$ (c) $9\frac{2}{3}$ (d) $11\frac{3}{16}$

Practice Set IV - 6

(a) $\frac{1}{3}$ (b) $\frac{1}{6}$ (c) $\frac{7}{11}$ (d) $\frac{1}{2}$

Practice Set IV - 7

(a) $\frac{3}{8}$ (b) $\frac{1}{8}$ (c) $\frac{1}{6}$ (d) $\frac{5}{16}$ (e) $\frac{7}{32}$ (f) $\frac{1}{32}$ (g) $\frac{7}{20}$

(h) $\frac{4}{15}$ (i) $2\frac{1}{4}$ (j) $1\frac{5}{8}$ (k) $\frac{3}{5}$ (l) $\frac{5}{6}$ (m) 1 (n) 1

Practice Set IV - 8

(a) $3\frac{3}{8}$ (b) $4\frac{1}{8}$ (c) $3\frac{1}{8}$ (d) $4\frac{1}{4}$ (e) $1\frac{1}{6}$

(f) $7\frac{3}{20}$ (g) $9\frac{1}{12}$ (h) $12\frac{7}{20}$ (i) $3\frac{7}{15}$ (j) $12\frac{1}{4}$

Practice Set IV - 9

(a) $\frac{11}{15}$ (b) $2\frac{7}{8}$ (c) $1\frac{1}{2}$ (d) $\frac{7}{8}$ (e) $1\frac{21}{22}$

(f) $15\frac{1}{2}$ (g) $7\frac{1}{5}$ (h) $\frac{13}{18}$ (i) $\frac{13}{20}$ (j) $8\frac{1}{2}$

Practice Set IV - 10

(a) $\frac{1}{9}$ (b) 1 (c) $\frac{1}{20}$ (d) $\frac{1}{30}$ (e) $2\frac{13}{18}$

Chapter 4 Review

(a) $\frac{15}{17}$ (b) $1\frac{7}{17}$ (c) $1\frac{11}{16}$ (d) $20\frac{1}{18}$ (e) $\frac{3}{20}$ (f) $2\frac{23}{56}$ (g) $12\frac{43}{60}$ (h) $\frac{19}{20}$
(i) $1\frac{71}{72}$ (j) $5\frac{11}{12}$ (k) 1 (l) $\frac{5}{24}$ (m) $7\frac{31}{60}$ (n) $7\frac{9}{10}$ (o) $\frac{23}{24}$ (p) $\frac{1}{3}$
(q) $1\frac{2}{9}$ (r) $3\frac{8}{9}$ (s) $3\frac{11}{14}$ (t) $7\frac{5}{9}$ (u) $16\frac{1}{6}$ (v) $\frac{5}{24}$ (w) 0 (x) $6\frac{7}{12}$

Practice Set V - 1

(a) .9 (b) .3 (c) .25 (d) .0009 (e) .012 (f) .022 (g) .5 (h) .032

Practice Set V - 2

(a) .172 (b) .094 (c) .625 (d) .313 (e) .25 (f) .125 (g) .078 (h) .5
(i) 1.375 (j) 1.438 (k) .75 (l) .875 (m) 2.625 (n) .038 (o) 1.141

Practice Set V - 3

(a) $\frac{3}{50}$ (b) $\frac{1}{4}$ (c) $\frac{99}{200}$ (d) $\frac{33}{100}$ (e) $\frac{63}{100}$ (f) $\frac{9}{1000}$ (g) $\frac{3}{10}$ (h) $\frac{751}{2000}$ (i) $1\frac{47}{250}$

Practice Set V - 4

(a) 25.108 (b) 34.45 (c) 11.2615 (d) 2052.2608 (e) 3.605 (f) 5.406 (g) 22.506
(h) 1014.89 (i) .0883 (j) 105.28 (k) 17.73 (l) 6.598 (m) 2.8 (n) 9

Practice Set V - 5

(a) 91.75 (b) 189.23 (c) 10,998.92 (d) 9.71 (e) 9.2869 (f) 2.647 (g) .0242 (h) .34168

Practice Set V - 6

(a) 1.40 (b) 37.6 (c) .1414 (d) 64.0 (e) .049764

Practice Set V - 7

(a) 105 (b) 53.928 (c) .3216 (d) .4648 (e) 2388.33 (f) .0684 (g) .0066091
(h) 556.22 (i) 800.46873 (j) 1.19275 (k) $148.48 (l) $652.96 (m) $576.24 (n) $38.08
(o) $27.90

Practice Set V - 8

(a) 36 (b) 5400 (c) 47 (d) 961 (e) 2450 (f) 71

Practice Set V - 9

(a) 30 (b) 500 (c) 150 (d) 800 (e) 80 (f) 800

Practice Set V - 10

(a) .26 (b) .21 (c) .057625 (d) .03 (e) .22 (f) .07 (g) .021 (h) 3.01 (i) 6.76 (j) 2.05

Practice Set V - 11

1) 10891 2) 127.5 3) 32.4 4) 144 5) 64 6) 4.9 7) 303.4 8) 11330 9) 100100 10) 184.9 11) 80
12) 301 13) 67.6 14) 136.47

Practice Set V - 12

(1) see text (2) see text (3) 34.3 (4) 3, 430 (5) 343 (6) .0343 (7) 3430
(8) .00343 (9) 3.43 (10) .343 (11) .0343 (12) 3.43 (13) 34, 300 (14) .343
(15) 3.43 (16) .0343 (17) .00343 (18) .000343 (19) 343 (20) 343 (21) 34.3
(22) 3.43 (23) 3.43 (24) .00343 (25) .0000343 (26) 3.43 (27) .0000343
(28) .00000343 (29) .00343 (30) 3.43 (31) 343 (32) 34.3 (33) .000343 (34) .343
(35) .00343 (36) .0343

Practice Set V - 13

I. (a) .9828 (b) 82.81 (c) 23.814 (d) .7488 (e) 39.6381 (f) 4.582833 (g) 1.2288
(h) 672.8176 (i) 2.02608 (j) .17024 (k) .13792 (l) 23.622 (m) 10.76154 (n) .680493
(o) 15.65541 (p) 4.5632 (q) 5.25 (r) 15.7552 (s) 18.48 (t) .18864 (u) 60.7087
(v) 475.41 (w) 1078 (x) 9823 (y) 1.4887 (z) .2273 (aa) .0171 (bb) .001289

II. (a) 900 (b) 2.098701299 (c) 2 (d) 7.530534351 (e) 2.9204 (f) 3 (g) .0405
(h) 123.1 (i) 100.5 (j) 80 (k) 9 (l) 9.1 (m) 5 (n) 2 (o) 20.2
(p) 71.42857143 (q) .4263 (r) .3655 (s) .0983525 (t) 83.59 (u) 835.9 (v) 8359
(w) 540 (x) 818.6667

Practice Set V - 14

1) 31420 2) .3142 3) 31.42 4) 3142 5) .3142 6) 3, 142, 000 7) .03142 8) 3.142
9) .003142 10) 3,142,000

Practice Set V - 15

(a) 2310; 23.1	(b) .2001; 2, 010, 000	(c) 48, 236; .048236	(d) .0231; 231
(e) 469.1; .04691	(f) 96, 390; .09639	(g) .08569; 8, 569, 000	(h) .0098751; 9875.1
(i) 187.54; 1.8754	(j) 91040; 9.104	(k) 876, 120; .876120	(l) 9.5431; 9, 543, 100
(m) 0.0998; 9.98	(n) .057624; 5, 762, 400	(o) .051; 510	(p) 79.99; 79.99
(q) 853, 330; .0085333	(r) .94999; 9499.9	(s) .087666; 8766.6	(t) .087632; 87632
(u).0099433; 994, 330	(v) 86432; 864.32	(w) 999, 990; .0099999	(x) .087432; 87432
(y).087432; 8743.2	(z) .095411; 9, 541, 100	(aa) 8765.4; .87654	

Practice Set V - 16

(a) .873 (b) .790 (c) .778 (d) .631 (e) .621 (f) .733
(a) .65 (b) .67 (c) .37 (d) .98 (e) .43 (f) .64

Practice Set V - 17

(a) 7.43 (b) .08 (c) 2.09 (d) .02 (e) 4.76 (f) .62 (g) 18.20 (h) .03 (i) 3600
(j) 1647.14 (k) .33 (l) .67
(a) 550.723 (b) 13.859 (c) 26.197 (d) 12.567 (e) 2.913 (f) 3.165 (g) 32.411 (h) 24.675 (i) 2.183
(j) 2.64 (k) 3.692 (l) .143

Practice Set V - 18

A:

(a) 590 (b) 0.0033 (c) 1760 (d) 0.8 (e) 1600 (f) 0.85 (g) 1910 (h) 0.0 (i) 1070
(j) 1.98 (k) 50 (l) 4.5 (m) 1430 (n) 1.43 (o) 876, 900 (p) 8.6 (q) 4, 900, 000 (r) 0.03

B:

(a) 1×10^5 or 10^5 (b) 1×10^2 (c) 10^6 (d) 10^{-4} (e) 10^{-8}
(f) 10^{-2} (g) 10^{-10} (h) 10^{-6} (i) 10^3 (j) 10^7

C:

a) 1, 000, 000 b) 10, 000 c) 1000 d) 10, 000, 000 e) .001 f) .00001 g) .01 h) .000001 i) 100

Practice Set V - 19

(a) 20, 000 (b) 8, 400, 000 (c) .0033 (d) 33 (e) .0000000847
(f) 3.5×10^{-4} (g) 8.39×10^{-4} (h) 1.0857×10^{4} (i) 8,769,000,000 (j) 0.0004235
(k) .0000006798 (l) 2.4681×10^{5} (m) 3.57×10^{-3} (n) 0.00008276 (o) .0000075
(p) 1.5×10^{-7} or 0.000015 (q) 40, 000, 000 (r) 4.36×10^{-5} (s) 4.5789×10^{4}
(t) 2.57×10^{2} (u) 8.32467×10^{3} (v) 26, 900 (w) 3.57×10^{-3} (x) 5×10^{-5}
(y) 4.83×10^{0} (z) 10^{-5}

Fraction Review

1:

(a) $4\frac{1}{27}$ (b) $10\frac{35}{64}$ (c) $20\frac{1}{12}$ (d) $25\frac{13}{24}$ (e) $2\frac{21}{40}$

2:

(a) $\frac{3}{4}$ (b) $\frac{10}{12}$ (c) $\frac{5}{6}$ (d) $\frac{1}{6}$ (e) $\frac{3}{4}$
(f) $\frac{9}{10}$ (g) $\frac{2}{3}$ (h) $\frac{5}{11}$

3:

(a) 4 (b) $3\frac{1}{5}$ (c) $8\frac{1}{3}$ (d) $1\frac{1}{12}$ (e) 3
(f) $9\frac{1}{3}$ (g) 14 (h) $4\frac{3}{4}$ (i) 9 (j) $3\frac{1}{2}$

4:

(a) $\frac{5}{18}$ (b) $6\frac{13}{32}$ (c) $15\frac{5}{12}$ (d) $\frac{7}{45}$ (e) $10\frac{23}{25}$ (f) $\frac{66}{125}$ (g) $4\frac{13}{16}$ (h) $16\frac{4}{5}$
(i) $1\frac{1}{2}$ (j) $\frac{5}{18}$ (k) $1\frac{1}{4}$ (l) $\frac{3}{10}$ (m) $31\frac{11}{16}$ (n) $\frac{9}{10}$ (o) $21\frac{21}{25}$ (p) $\frac{1}{2}$
(q) $10\frac{11}{36}$ (r) $812\frac{1}{2}$

5:

(a) $\frac{5}{8}$ (b) $3\frac{1}{5}$ (c) $10\frac{1}{3}$ (d) $\frac{3}{10}$ (e) 12
(f) $\frac{3}{10}$ (g) $\frac{3}{16}$ (h) $8\frac{1}{4}$ (i) $58\frac{13}{15}$ (j) $\frac{3}{4}$

6:

(a) $431\frac{1}{4}$ (b) $\frac{4}{21}$ (c) $2\frac{18}{55}$ (d) $3\frac{9}{31}$ (e) $\frac{3}{10}$
(f) $\frac{3}{10}$ (g) $72\frac{2}{3}$ (h) $1\frac{13}{29}$ (i) 2

Practice Set VI - 1

(a)	A	α	**alpha**
(b)	B	β	beta
(c)	Π	π	**pi**
(d)	Γ	γ	**gamma**
(e)	Σ	σ	**sigma**
(f)	M	μ	mu
(g)	Θ	θ	theta
(h)	Ω	ω	omega
(i)	Δ	δ	delta
(j)	Λ	λ	**lambda**

Practice Set VI - 2

(a) parallel
(b) right; perpendicular
(c) (i) eccentric (ii) concentric
(d) (A) plunger (B) barrel (C) tip (D) eccentrically
(e) 360
(f) (i) 45° (ii) 30° (iii) 180°

Practice Set VI - 3

(a) meniscus (b) capillary action (c) parallax
(d) mass per unit volume (e) 1 g/cc ; 62.4 lbs/ft^3 (f) comparison of densities to the density of water

Practice Set VII - 1

(1) .15 (2) .33 (3) .40 (4) .01 (5) .09 (6) 1.25 (7) .943 (8) 1 (9) .05

Practice Set VII - 2

(1) 10% (2) 12% (3) 12.5% (4) 9% (5) 630% (6) 76.2%
(7) 87.5% (8) 225% (9) 90% (10) 37.5% (11) 8.5% (12) 10%

Practice Set VII - 3

(1) $\frac{3}{5}$ (2) $\frac{1}{2}$ (3) $\frac{1}{10}$ (4) $\frac{2}{25}$ (5) $1\frac{1}{10}$ (6) $\frac{9}{10}$

Pracitce Set VII - 4

(1) 25% (2) 60% (3) 70% (4) $8.\bar{3}\%$ (5) 18.75% (6) 87.5% (7) $83.\bar{3}\%$ (8) 20%

Practice Set VII - 5

1. (1) .025 (2) .085 (3) .0711 (4) .0625 (5) .095 (6) 1.90
2. (7) 33% (8) 36.33% (9) 98.7% (10) 63% (11) 11% (12) 1637.5%
3. (13) 12.5% (14) 62.5% (15) 14.3% (16) 57.1% (17) 11.1% (18) 55.6% (19) 9.1% (20) 63.6%
4. (21) $\frac{1}{50}$ (22) $\frac{2}{25}$ (23) $\frac{1}{5}$ (24) $\frac{2}{5}$ (25) $\frac{8}{25}$ (26) $\frac{12}{25}$ (27) $\frac{77}{200}$ (28) $\frac{7}{400}$
5. (29) 8%; .08; $\frac{2}{25}$ (30) 7.5%; .075; $\frac{3}{40}$ (31) 92.5%; .925; $\frac{37}{40}$
   (32) 66.7%; .667; $\frac{667}{1000}$ (33) 42.86%; .4286; $\frac{3}{7}$ (34) 12.5%; .125; $\frac{1}{8}$
   (35) 65, 000%; 650; 650 (36) 56.25%; .5625; $\frac{9}{16}$ (37) 125%; 1.25; $1\frac{1}{4}$
   (38) 26.19%; .2619; $\frac{11}{42}$ (39) 33.3%; .333; $\frac{333}{1000}$ (40) 362.5%; 3.625; $3\frac{5}{8}$
   (41) 155.56%; 1.5556; $1\frac{5}{9}$ (42) 3.25%; .0325; $\frac{13}{400}$

Practice Set VII - 6

(1) 50 (2) 500 (3) 50 (4) 75 (5) 300 (6) 30.006
(7) 111 (8) 60 (9) 166.5 (10) 100 (11) 450 (12) 480

Practice Set VII - 7

1. \$705 2. 33.75 lbs 3. \$465.80 4. 410 ml

Practice Set VII - 8

1. 29.63% 2. 2.05% 3. 10% 4. 8% 5. 15.6% 6. 8.3% 7. 8.125% 8. 22.92% 9. 70.8% 10. 11.9%

Practice Set VII - 9

1. \$5.83 2. \$9.50 3. \$5.28 4. \$3.62 5. \$7.75

Practice Set VII - 10

1. a. 4.48 b. 900 c. 160 d. 5.44 e. 112.7 f. 10.14 g. .0325 h. 7.25
2. a. 307.5 sq ft b. 1537.5 sq ft

Practice Set VII - 11

Company A	Company B
$4.76	$4.78
$6.47	$6.72
$5.50	$5.38
$5.91	$5.97
$1.56	$1.83
$4.06	$3.78
$3.32	$3.23
$46.80	$45.96
$1.86	$2.07
$3.74	$3.82
$1.99	$1.88

Practice Set VII - 12

(1) 14g% (2) 0.9g% (3) 0.5g% (4) 1g% (5) 18g/100ml (6) 9 g/100 ml
(7) 0.003 g / 100 ml (8) 4.5 g / 100 ml (9) 0.85 g/100 ml (10) 4g% (11) 3.2 mg%
(12) 0.4mg% (13) 0.1 mg/100 ml (14) 17 mg/ 100 ml

Practice Set VII - 13

1. a. 12g% b. $7.\bar{3}$g% c. 8g% d. 14g% e. 10g% f. 16g%
2. a. 0.9% b. 5% c. 4.5% d. 10% e. 2% f. 1% g. 70% h. 2% i. 9%
3. a. 23.7% b. 237% c. 2370% d. 23, 700% e. 2.37% f. .237% g. .0237% h. .45 i. .001
   j. 0.4327 k. 0.0832 l. 0.09372 m. 0.003271 n. 0.0016137

Practice Set VIII - 1

(a) 2:1 (b) 40:80 = 1:2 (c) 12:5 (d) 70:29 (e) 29:1

Practice Set VIII -2

(a) $\frac{1}{3}$ (b) $\frac{1}{9}$ (c) $\frac{1}{3}$ (d) $\frac{1}{2}$ (e) $\frac{1}{8}$ (f) $\frac{9}{10}$

Practice Set VIII - 3

(a) 5 g : 100 ml ; 1 g : 20 ml (b) 10 mg : 1 ml (c) 100 mg : 1 cc (d) 1 ml : 100 lbs
(e) 25 mg : 1 ml (f) 0.1 mg : 2.0 kg or 1 mg : 20 kg (g) 1 cc : 5 lb

Practice Set VIII - 4

(a) 20 (b) 3 (c) 1.5 (d) 17 (e) 40 (f) 2 (g) 1000 (h) 3
(i) 9 (j) 56 (k) 0.40 (l) 2 (m) 400 (n) 6 (o) $\frac{1}{100}$

Practice Set VIII - 5

(a) 30 ml (b) 20 cc (c) 0.4 cc (d) 70 mg

Practice Set VIII - 6

(a) 1 (b) 5 (c) 1 (d) 7.875 (e) 1.125 (f) 3.889 (g) 27 (h) 6.667 (i) 1.5 (j) 6.286 (k) 100
(l) 10.417 (m) 10.769 (n) 2 (o) 27 (p) 2.9 (q) 15 (r) 1.944 cc (s) 7 cc (t) 3.5 cc (u) 13 cc

Chapter 8 Review

(a) 1.875 mg (b) 7 drops (c) 7 ml (d) 5.5 ml (e) 15 cc (f) 2.32 cc (g) 20 g (h) 9 g
(i) 4 cc (j) 17 mg (k) 6 drops (l) 2.75 mg (m) 1.375 mg (n) 20 g (o) 8 cc (p) 300 cc
(q) 6.25 mg (r) 4.8 drops (s) 13 ml (t) 3.5 mg (u) 0.175 cc (v) 32 mg (w) 3.2 ml (x) 50 mg
(y) 60 mg (z) 5 cc (aa) 0.833 ml (bb)0.52 ml (cc) 0.75 mg (dd) 0.9 ml (ee) 4.25 mg (ff) .36 cc
(gg) 3.25 mg (hh) 4.2 cc (ii) 0.575 cc (jj) 0.4 ml

Practice Set IX - 1

(a) 5 cc (b) 13.4 cc (c) 160 mg (d) 16 tabs (e) 150 mg (f) 1.5 cc (g) 20 g (h) 6 g
(i) 60 g (j) 9 g; 0.9 g (k) 30 g; 1.5 g; 101 g; 15.5 g (l) 20 cages (m) $171 (n) 6.25 cc

Practice Set IX - 2

(a) 2.55 cc (b) 2.52 cc (c) 1.5 cc (d) 75 cc (e) 16.7 cc

Practice Set IX - 3

(a) 360 g (b) 200 g (c) 25 g (d) 50 g (e) 150 ml (f) 400 ml
(g) 6 g; 12 g (h) 32 ml (i) 2.25 g (j) 0.75 g (k) 1 g (l) 0.4 g

Practice Set IX - 4

(a) (i) 3 cc (ii) 13 cc (b) (i) 5 cc (ii) 21.7 cc (c) (i) 0.6 cc (ii) 2.6 cc (d) (i) 180 mg (ii) 1.8 cc
(e) 1.4 ml (f) (i) 11.25 mg (ii) 1 tab (g) (i) 187.5 mg (ii) 7.5 cc (h) 4167 WBC (i) 5.3 cc

Practice Set IX - 5

(a) 1.4 cc (b) (i) 1.2 (ii) 1.8 (iii) 14.6 (iv) 7 (v) 3.6 (c) (i) 2 (ii) 3 (iii) 24.3 (iv) 11.7 (v) 6
(d) (i) 0.9 (ii) 1.275 (iii) 2.7 (iv) 1.95 (v) 6.75 (e) (i) 9 (ii) 31.25 (iii) 6.25 (iv) 18.25 (v) 4.5
(f) (i) 54 (ii) 187.5 (iii) 37.5 (iv) 109.5 (v) 27 (g) (i) 3.6 (ii) 12.5 (iii) 2.5 (iv) 7.3 (v) 1.8

Practice Set IX - 6

(a) (i) 7 cc (ii) 4.2 cc (iii) 2.8 cc (b) (i) 9.4 cc; (ii) 5.64 cc (iii) 3.8 cc (c) (i) 3 cc (ii) 1.8 cc (iii) 1.2 cc

Practice Set IX - 7

1. (a) 22.5 g (b) 10.5 ml (c) 32.5 ml (d) 47.5 g (e) 325 ml (f) 0.675 g
   (g) 1/4 g (h) 0.95 g (i) 20 g (j) 0.75 g (k) 0.35 g
2. (a) 95% (b) 0.9% (c) 2% (d) 5% (e) 0.9% (f) 3% (g) 70%

Practice Set IX - 8

(1) 3.8 cc (2) 8.3 cc (3) 0.45 cc (4) 2.1 cc (5) 1.2 ml (6) 9.75 mg; 1 tab (7) 37.5 mg; 1.5 cc
(8) 7.5 cc (9) 2 cc (10) 12.4 cc (11) 18 g (12) 29.5 g (13) 0.765 g
(14) 1/2 g (15) 0.95 g (16) 1.95 cc (17) 10.4 cc (18) 9.6 cc (19) 13.3 cc

Practice Set X - 1

(a) hecto- (b) deci- (c) none (d) kilo- (e) milli- (f) deka- (g) centi-

Practice Set X - 2

(a) km; 1,000 m (b) dm; $^1/_{10}$ m (c) mg; $^1/_{1000}$ g (d) dkg; 10 g (e) m; 1 meter (f) dl; $^1/_{10}$ L
(g) dkm; 10 m (h) g; 1 g ram (i) hm; 100 m (j) dg; $^1/_{10}$ g (k) cl; $^1/_{100}$ L (l) l; 1 liter
(m) dkl; 10 L (n) hl; 100 L (o) kl; 1000 L (p) ml; $^1/_{1000}$ L (q) cm; $^1/_{100}$ m

Practice Set X - 3

(a) 1200 dm (b) 12, 000 mg (c) 2100 cl (d) 15 mm (e) 5510 cg (f) 61, 250 mg
(g) 3000 L (h) 40, 100 cl (i) 5, 151, 200 ml (j) 12, 140 km (k) 0.112 dg (l) 0.00021 kl
(m) 0.0123 m (n) 0.051 kg (o) 0.0235 dkm (p) 0.653 hl (q) 0.0034 km (r) 0.635 dkm
(s) 0.1511235 kl

Practice Set XI - 1

1) pt 2) pound 3) ounce 4) yd 5) in 6) Tablespoon 7) teaspoon 8) fl oz
9) gal 10) ft 11) c 12) mi 13) oz 14) quart 15) gr

Practice Set XI - 2

a. 9 b. 2 c. 18 d. 54 e. 10 f. 40 g. 27 h. 13
i. 108 j. 168 k. 27,000 l. 48 m. 10,560 n. 3400 o. 9 p. 1.5625

Practice Set XI - 3

a. 1 b. 2; 1 c. 8; 4; 1 d. 12; 24; 384 e. 1 f. 48 g. 72 h. 12 i. $^{7}/_{12}$
j. 4.5 k. 2/3 l. 3 m. $^{1}/_{3}$ n. 180 o. 60 p. $^{1}/_{2}$ q. 384 r. 30

Practice Set XI - 4

a. 1 b. 16 c. 1-$^{1}/_{2}$ d. 6 e. 24 f. 1-$^{1}/_{8}$ g. 4 h. 8 i. 8 j. 32,000
k. $^{1}/_{6}$ l. 1.95 m. 2-$^{1}/_{2}$ n. 1.09375 o. 2 p. 24 q. 4 r. $^{3}/_{8}$ s. 9.6
t. 7 u. 3 v. 2 w. 9 x. 5 y. 1 z. 2-$^{1}/_{2}$ aa. 80 bb. 20

Practice Set XII - 1

(a) 7 (b) 12.5 (c) 2.7 (d) 1.59 (e) 45 (f) 908
(g) 1-$^{1}/_{8}$ (h) 105 (i) 45 (j) 0.04 (k) 59.4 (l) 118.2

Practice Set XII - 2

a. 104°F b. 15.6°C c. 98.6°F d. 18.3°C e. 0° f. 21.1°C g. 7.2°C
h. 22.8°C i. 37.8°C j. 25.6°C k. –17.8°C l. 176°F m. –40° n. 212°F
o. –23.3°C p. 26.7°C q. 77°F r. 122°F s. –12.°C2 t. 64.4°F

Practice Set XII - 3

a. 45 b. 141.5 c. 2.2 d. 127.35 e. 84.9 f. 7 g. 113.5 h. 0.44 i. 600 j. 240
k. 20 l. 1500 m. 3.750 n. 3 o. 30 p. 0.8 q. 1.6 r. 1.8 s. 3-$^{1}/_{3}$ t. 15
u. 45 v. 2.5 w. 17 x. 5-$^{2}/_{3}$ y. 3 z. $^{1}/_{10}$ aa. 0.2 bb. 5 cc. 0.9 dd. 14.7

Practice Set XII - 4

a. 2 b. 9 c. 2 d. 2 e. 40 f. 4000 g. 2 h. 24 i. 6 j. 6
k. 3 l. 8 m. 1 n. 84.9 o. 2/3 p. 180 q. 1 r. 83.33 s. 2 t. 25
u. 12 v. 1.4 w. 1/5 x. 5 y. 3 z. 2.5 aa. 3-1/4 bb. 1.6 cc. 2.4 dd. 5.1
ee. 0.8 ff. 2 gg. 1-1/2 hh. 1-1/2 ii. 141.5 jj. 192 kk. 60 ll. 25 mm. 105 nn. 7.5

Practice Set XII - 5

a. 5 b. 1000 c. 1; 1/2; 500 d. 1/2 e. 1/2 f. 2500; 2500 g. 250 h. 100
i. 30 j. 32 k. 15 l. 1000; 2; 1 m. 1 n. 60 o. 180 p. 4.4
q. 0.15 r. 60 s. 4; 8; 4000 t. 8000 u. 500 v. 0.6 w. 1/4 x. 1
y. 1500 z. 24.2 aa. 1 bb. 1 cc. 30 dd. 1 ee. 2

Practice Set XIII - 1

(a) see text (b) 0.7 ml (c) 32 ml (d) 1.5 gal/day; 6 gals for 4 days
(e) 1000 mg; 5 ml (f) up to 11, 000 ml over 24 hours (g) 2200 mg; 44 ml
(h) 12 bolus per dose; 36 bolus for 6 days

Practice Set XIII - 2

(a) (i) 12.5 mg (ii) 1.25 ml (b) (i) 36 mg (ii) 0.9 ml (c) (i) 40 mg (ii) 0.8 ml (iii) 8 ml
(d) (i) 3 caps (ii) 21 caps (e) (i) 0.19 cc (ii) 0.08 cc (f) (i) 0.03 cc (ii) 0.04 cc
(g) (i) 0.12 ml (ii) 0.12 ml

Practice Set XIII - 3

(1) (i) 20.5 ml (ii) 6.8 cc (iii) 10 cc (iv) 37.7 cc
(2) (a)(i) 0.55 cc (ii) 0.77 cc (iii) 2.8 cc (2)(b)(i) 0.17 cc (ii) 0.11 cc (iii) 0.39 ml
(2) (c)(i) 2.2 cc (ii) 1.5 cc (iii) 4.0 cc (3) (i) 4.4 ml (ii) 2.9 ml (iii) 20 ml (iv) 1 ml

Practice Set XIV - 1

(a) 1.75 L; 0.75 L water (b) 2.2 1 L; 0.79 water (c) 2.4 L; 9.6 L (d) 3750 ml; 3675 ml water
(e) 2000 ml; 1980 ml (f) 1388.9 ml; 1111.1 ml (g) 2.1 L; 0.9 (h) 3.68 L; 1.32 L
(i) 4200 ml; 3500 ml (j) 3 L; 27 L (k) 4 L of each

Practice Set XIV - 2

(a)(i) 1.5 L; 28.5 L water (ii) 0.3 L; 29.7 L (b) 600 ml; 5.4 L (c)(i) 5.7 L stock; 0.3 L water
(ii) 6.63 L stock and 2.37 L water (d) 166.7 ml stock; 833.3 ml H_2O (e) 2.1 gals stock; 0.9 gal water
(f) 28.6 L; 8.57 L (g) 7200 ml; 7000 ml (h) 2.5 L stock; 22.5 L H_2O
(i) 15 L each; 3L stock + 27 L H_2O

Practice Set XIV - 3

(1) 700 ml (2) 2.95 L (3) 3 L (3000 ml) (4) 2 L (5) 2.5 L (6) 5 L (7) 2500 ml (8) 1 L

Practice Set XIV - 4

(1) 1.4 gal; 0.6 gal water (2) 3600 ml; 3500 ml (3) 1.5 L stock; 13.5 L H_2O
(4) 10 L each; 2 L stock + 18 L H_2O (5) (i) 1 L stock + 19 L H_2O (ii) 0.2 L stock + 19.8 L H_2O
(6) 1/2 L stock + 4.5 L H_2O (7) (i) 4.74 L stock + 0.26 L H_2O (ii) 5.2 L + 1.8 L

Practice Set XV - 1

1.	2.	3.
0.032	graph	110
0.044		225
0.03		335
0.018		390
0.022		300
0.048		200

Practice Set XV - 2

1.

A	(1,1)	H	(0,3)
B	(2.4,2.4)	I	(8,2.2)
C	(3.4,0)	J	(0.4, −0.6)
D	(2, −1.6)	K	(6.1,0.8)
E	(4.6, −1.2)	L	(8.6, −1)
F	(5,1.6)	M	(5.8,2.4)
G	(6.6, −3)	N	(6, −1)

2.

	Time	millivolts
A	1.4 sec	1.6
B	2.4 sec	0.8
C	7.8 sec	2.6
D	8.8 sec	0.6
E	13.8 sec	1.4
F	14.6 sec	0.8
G	14.8 sec	0.4
H	16.2 sec	0.6
I	19.6 sec	1.0
J	19.6 sec	2.2
K	20.4 sec	0.6

Practice Set XVI - 1

1. (a) 28 (b) 5.6 (c) 190 (d) 0 (e) 33.2
2. (a) 50 (b) 630 (c) 534

Practice Set XVI - 2

1. (a) T (b) T (c) T (d) F (e) F (f) T (g) F (h) T (i) T (j) T (k) F
2. (l) b (m) c (n) d (o) b

Practice Set XVI - 3

1. (a) 11 (b) 17.67 (c) 3.24
2. (a) mean: 67 median: 64.5 mode: 60 (b) 8.21